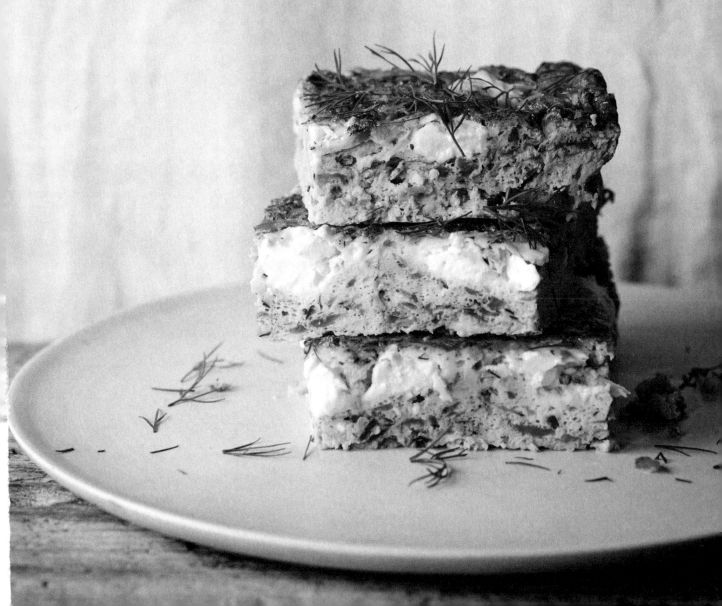

FAST FOOD,
GOOD FOOD

Also by Andrew Weil, MD

True Food

Spontaneous Happiness

You Can't Afford to Get Sick: Your Guide to Optimum Health and Health Care
(originally published as *Why Our Health Matters*)

Integrative Oncology
(with Donald Abrams, MD)

Healthy Aging: A Lifelong Guide to Your Well-Being

The Healthy Kitchen: Recipes for a Better Body, Life, and Spirit
(with Rosie Daley)

Eating Well for Optimum Health: The Essential Guide to Food, Diet, and Nutrition

Eight Weeks to Optimum Health: A Proven Program for Taking Advantage
of Your Body's Natural Healing Power

Spontaneous Healing: How to Discover and Enhance Your Body's Natural Ability
to Maintain and Heal Itself

Natural Health, Natural Medicine: The Complete Guide to Wellness and
Self-Care for Optimum Health

Health and Healing

From Chocolate to Morphine: Everything You Need to Know About Mind-Altering Drugs
(with Winifred Rosen)

The Marriage of the Sun and Moon: Dispatches from
the Frontiers of Consciousness

The Natural Mind: A Revolutionary Approach to the Drug Problem

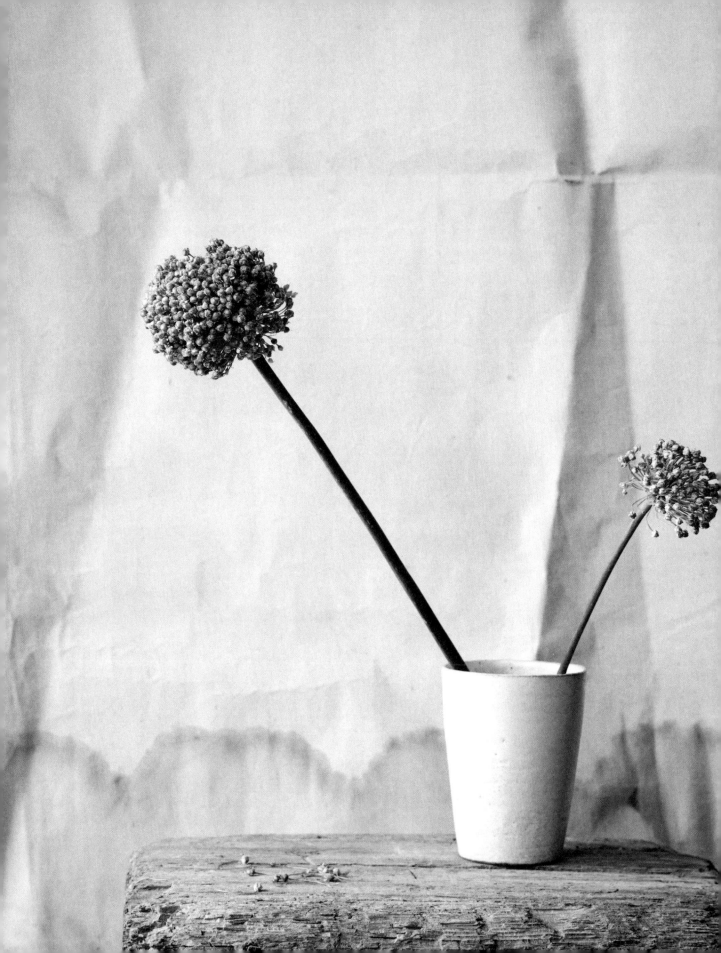

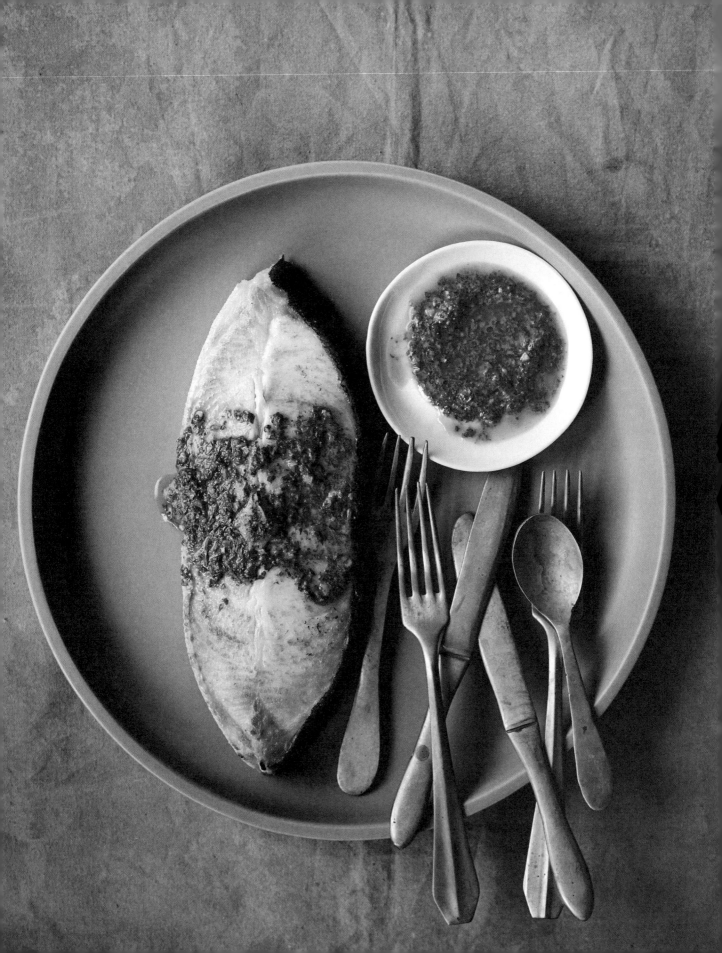

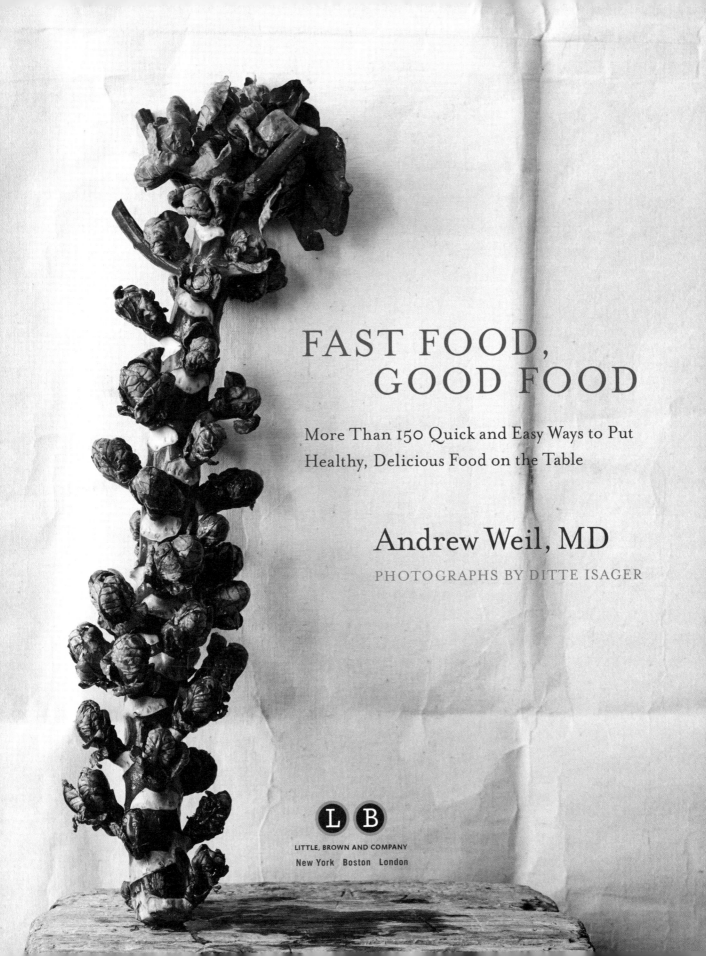

FAST FOOD, GOOD FOOD

More Than 150 Quick and Easy Ways to Put
Healthy, Delicious Food on the Table

Andrew Weil, MD

PHOTOGRAPHS BY DITTE ISAGER

L B

LITTLE, BROWN AND COMPANY

New York   Boston   London

Little, Brown and Company
Hachette Book Group
1290 Avenue of the Americas, New York NY 10104
littlebrown.com

First Edition: October 2015

Little, Brown and Company is a division of Hachette Book
Group, Inc. The Little, Brown name and logo are trademarks of
Hachette Book Group, Inc.

The publisher is not responsible for websites (or their content)
that are not owned by the publisher.

Book design by Gary Tooth / Empire Design Studio

Prop styling by Christine Rudolph
Food styling by Susie Theodorou

ISBN 978-0-316-32942-2
LCCN 2015931944

10 9 8 7 6 5 4 3 2 1

SC

Printed in China

CONTENTS

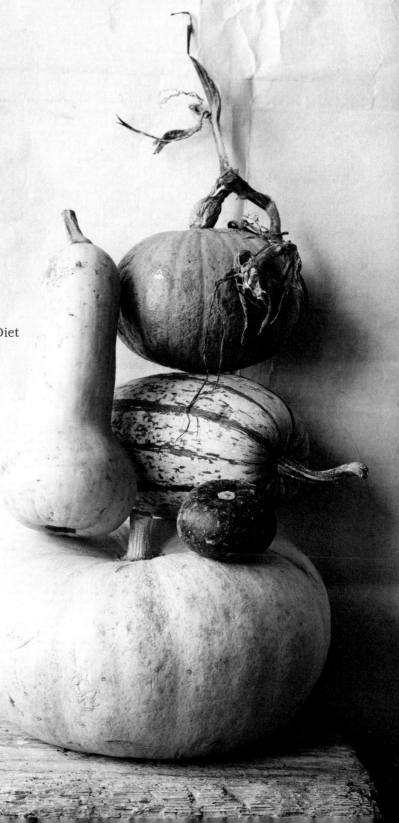

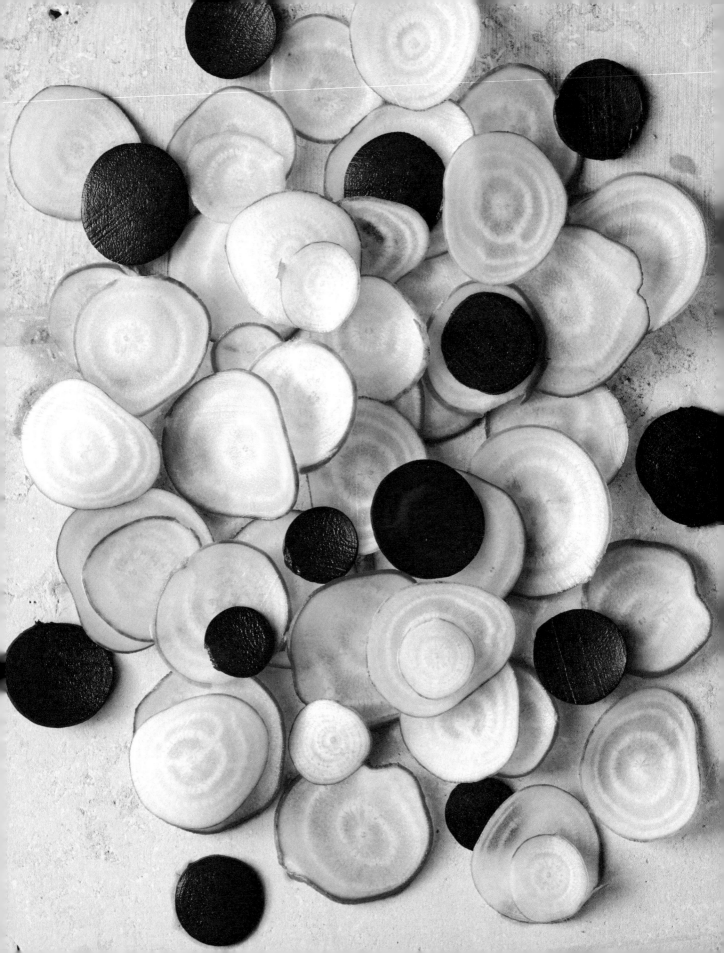

intro

INTRODUCTION

Sales of cookbooks are at an all-time high, as are the ratings of cooking shows on television. Yet fewer people than ever are cooking meals at home. What gives? Apparently, for book buyers and followers of the Food Network, cooking is nothing more than entertainment.

People say they don't have time to cook. Many also say they don't know how or lack the skills to reproduce dishes pictured in books and made by celebrity chefs on television. I love to cook, but I don't care to knock myself out in the kitchen. I enjoy simple meals that are quick and easy and use fresh ingredients of the best quality. I want those ingredients to shine, not be lost in fussy preparations. I go for bold flavors and visual appeal. Forget complicated recipes; cooking should be fun.

Popular Food Network shows portray cooking as competitive. I'd rather it be contemplative. That's why I got into it when I was a medical student. I discovered that imagining a wonderful meal and then making it for myself was the perfect way to get my mind back in balance after long stretches of working in depressing hospital wards where the only available food was wretched. Chopping vegetables became a welcome meditation. Getting a meal to come as close as possible to the way I imagined it was an exercise in practical magic.

Later, I learned the principles of good nutrition and the science of dietary influences on health, and I found it easy to apply that information to my cooking. I have always believed that delicious food and food that's good for us can be one and the same. Like most people, you have probably been served unsatisfying, possibly inedible "health food." Maybe you think that eating healthy means giving up everything you like. I assure you that is not so. The recipes in this book conform to cutting-edge nutritional science; they also yield dishes that taste great. As a practitioner of integrative medicine, which places great importance on lifestyle, and as an author of books on health, I want to see eating habits improve. But I know that, first and foremost, food has to taste great.

For at least ten years now I have recommended an anti-inflammatory diet for its power to optimize health and reduce risks of serious disease. (See page 279 for more.) Inflammation is useful, a cornerstone of the body's defensive and healing systems. It is also so powerful that it can be harmful if it persists or serves no purpose. A great deal of scientific evidence supports the idea that chronic, low-level, purposeless inflammation is the root cause of coronary artery disease, Alzheimer's disease, and many other conditions that kill or disable people prematurely. It also increases the risk of cancer, because inflammation and abnormal cell proliferation are closely linked.

Diet influences inflammation, and the mainstream diet in North America is clearly pro-inflammatory. The fats and carbohydrates that predominate in it favor inflammation, and it is deficient in the protective compounds found in vegetables, fruits, herbs, and spices. The first principle of the Anti-Inflammatory Diet is to eliminate refined, processed, and manufactured food. Do that, and you are well along the path to eating right for optimum health.

I used the Mediterranean diet as a template for my eating plan, because strong research data correlate it with longevity, good health, and the lowest overall disease risk. I added Asian influences to the basic Mediterranean diet—spices like ginger and turmeric, for example, which are potent natural anti-inflammatory agents. And I tweaked it in other ways to increase its potential to contain inappropriate inflammation.

Look at the Anti-Inflammatory Diet Pyramid on page 278 to get an overview of the nutritional philosophy underlying this book. Note that vegetables form its base and dark chocolate is at the very top. Olive oil has a strong midlevel position. I assure you that following the guidelines illustrated in the pyramid is not onerous, will not detract from the pleasure of eating, and will protect your long-term health and wellness.

The recipes in these pages are not difficult. They can be prepared quickly and they give results you will love. Keep in mind that recipes are made to be tinkered with. Feel free to experiment with them, changing ingredients to suit your taste. Above all: keep it simple. You will find many suggestions in the Pantry and Quick Tips and Basics sections to make your cooking easy and fun.

Note that recipes are designated *veg* for vegetarian, *v* for vegan, and *gf* for gluten-free. Those marked *veg**, *v**, and *gf** can be prepared as vegetarian, vegan, or gluten-free by substituting or omitting specific ingredients.

This book is about fast food in the best sense—real food that takes little time. Many recipes can be made in just thirty minutes. Some need more cooking time, but the preparation is quick. Others may require a lot of chopping but little cooking time. None are complicated or difficult. But do take time to enjoy your meals. One aspect of the good health associated with the Mediterranean diet is that people of the region do not eat mindlessly or on the run. They take pleasure in excellent food eaten without haste in the company of friends and family. I try to follow their example.

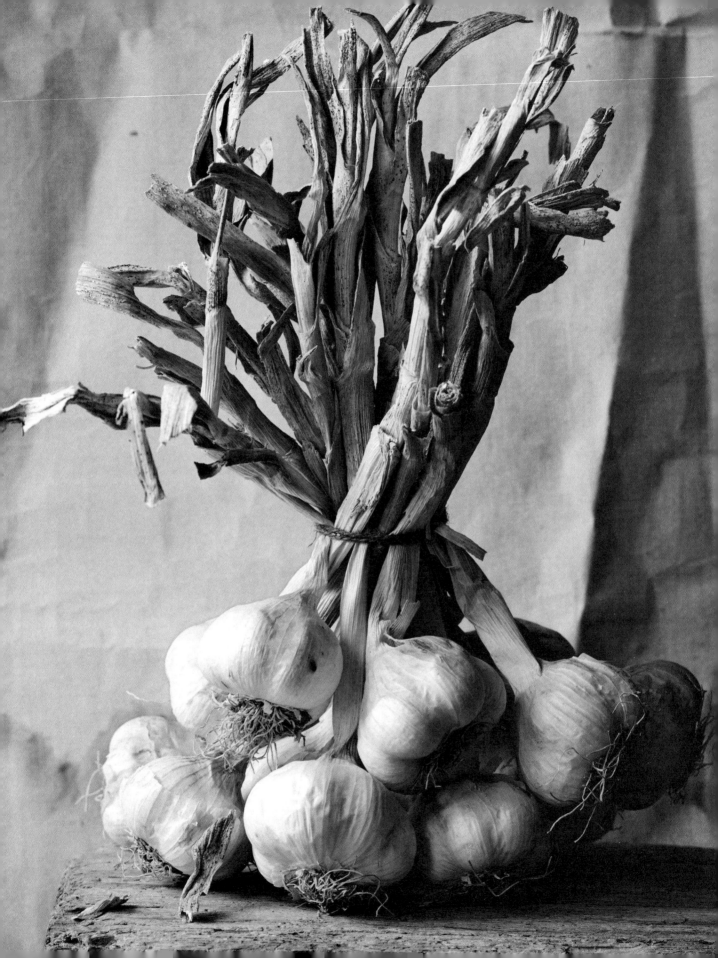

Pantry
Quick tips!

PANTRY ESSENTIALS

I like to keep a well-stocked pantry. It allows me to pull together a meal quickly and efficiently. Some of the ingredients I use may be unfamiliar, but I assure you that all can be found in supermarkets, Asian groceries, farmers' markets, or online.

ALMOND FLOUR: Made from raw, blanched almonds, this gluten-free product is useful in baking and a good source of protein and minerals as well as fat. It goes rancid quickly, so always give it a sniff test before using to make sure it's fresh (there should be no odor resembling that of oil paint), and store it in an airtight container in the freezer. Bob's Red Mill makes a good product; go to bobsredmill.com.

ASIAN INGREDIENTS: If you do not have a nearby Asian grocery store, it's easy to find all of the Asian ingredients called for in these recipes online. Look for sites selling specialty groceries, such as hmart.com (Korean foods), importfood.com (Thai), asianfoodgrocer.com (Japanese), and waiyeehong.com (Chinese).

BEANS: Canned beans allow you to make bean dishes quickly. Look for brands packed in water and salt only, with no additives, organic if possible. Trader Joe's has excellent organic canned great northern beans. Look for good-quality canned black beans and garbanzos in natural-food stores; I recommend Eden Foods brand.

BLACK PEPPER: Buy whole black peppercorns and grind them as needed in a pepper grinder. Some grinders allow you to adjust the particle size of the grains.

BREAD CRUMBS: Homemade bread crumbs are superior to packaged ones, although in a pinch, you can use Japanese-style panko bread crumbs, made from bread without crust. See Basics on page 274 for directions on making your own.

BUTTER: The latest research on the health effects of saturated fat indicates that it's not as bad as we used to think, and dairy fat may be the safest kind. Butter is used in this book in small amounts for flavor. Look for unsalted butter made from cream from grass-fed cows. A good brand is Kerrygold, made in Ireland and widely available in the United States and Canada; see kerrygoldusa.com/where-to-buy.

CHILIES: Many recipes in this book call for fresh or dried chilies. Pay attention to how much heat you and the people you cook for like and can tolerate; more chili can always be added at the table. Handle fresh chilies cautiously—use gloves if necessary—to avoid getting their juice on your skin or in your eyes. The greatest concentration of capsaicin, the compound responsible for pungency, is in the white pith to which seeds are attached. Removing it wholly or in part will tame a hot pepper. Choose fresh peppers with shiny, taut skin that is free of blemishes such as dark or soft spots. Dried chilies should be red or reddish brown.

CITRUS ZEST: The outer peel of citrus fruits—the zest—is rich in highly flavored oils that can brighten the taste of many dishes. Use zest only from organic oranges, lemons, and limes; conventionally grown citrus is likely to have agrichemical residues in the peel. The zest is best removed with a tool designed for that purpose or with a Microplane grater, but you can use a vegetable peeler too. Try not to take any of the bitter underlying white tissue.

DIJON MUSTARD: This strong condiment should be a light yellow-brown, with a pungent aroma. The best brands come from France. Once opened, a jar will keep in the refrigerator for a long time.

EDAMAME: Green soybeans, edamame are usually steamed in the pod, salted, and eaten hot or cold as a snack or appetizer. They are widely available, both fresh and frozen, either in the pod or shelled.

FARRO: Farro is an ancient variety of wheat. Pearled farro is partially hulled, and this greatly shortens the cooking time of the whole grains. It is available online and in many grocery stores. Farro contains gluten, but those with gluten sensitivity may find it more tolerable than common forms of wheat.

FISH: Omega-3-rich fish like salmon, sablefish, sardines, and mackerel are staples of the Anti-Inflammatory Diet. Sockeye salmon is a particularly good choice because it cannot be farmed and is less likely to be contaminated with toxins. The Monterey Bay Aquarium's Seafood Watch website (seafoodwatch.org/cr/seafoodwatch.aspx) is a useful consumer guide that rates fish and shellfish for both sustainability and toxic load.

FISH SAUCE: A staple of southeast Asian cooking, fish sauce is an intensely flavored condiment made from fermented fish (anchovies especially), salt, and water. The Vietnamese product, known as *nuoc mam*, is best, and Red Boat is a preferred, chemical-free brand, available in Asian food stores and online.

GARLIC: Choose heads of garlic with large, firm cloves. All the recipes in this book that call for garlic instruct you to mash the peeled cloves with a garlic press and let them sit, exposed to air, for at least ten minutes before adding them to a dish. This allows for the formation of allicin, the compound responsible for garlic's many health benefits. Store garlic at room temperature in an open container (such as a mesh basket), preferably in a dark place away from other foods.

GINGER: Select roots that are plump and firm. Peel what you need with a vegetable peeler and grate the root lengthwise with a Microplane grater or rasp. Store unpeeled ginger in a zip-top bag in the crisper drawer of the refrigerator.

GRAPESEED OIL: When you want a neutral flavor, grapeseed oil is best for sautéing. Buy expeller-pressed grapeseed oil. Once a bottle is opened, keep it in the refrigerator.

KASHA: Also known as buckwheat groats, this cracked grain comes raw or toasted. Buy the toasted variety.

KOMBU: A type of seaweed (kelp), kombu is used to flavor soups and broths, especially in Japanese cuisine. Do not rinse or wipe the dried strips before using them. Remove and discard them after simmering in liquid.

MAPLE SYRUP: This is my preferred sweetener, for its flavor and low fructose content. Many recipes in this book call for grade B maple syrup, which is best for cooking. When the syrup is used in small amounts, the maple flavor is not detectable. Store syrup in the refrigerator after opening. Grade A maple syrup is produced earlier in the season and has a lighter color and fewer minerals. It also has a more delicate maple flavor, which is why I recommend it for the flavored syrups on pages 275–77.

MEAT: Meat is used sparingly in the Anti-Inflammatory Diet, more as a special-occasion food than an everyday one. A few recipes in this book call for bison, which is preferable to beef and increasingly available. Choose grass-finished bison (that is, from animals that have foraged all their lives and have not been fattened on grain in feedlots before slaughter) raised without hormones or antibiotics. Grass-finished beef, raised without hormones or antibiotics, is an alternative.

MIRIN: A naturally sweet, traditional rice wine used in Japanese cooking. Look for hon-mirin ("true mirin") with an alcohol content of 12 percent. Takara is a good brand, available online from vendomestore.com and other sites. Eden Foods brand is also acceptable (edenfoods.com). Common commercial products are low in alcohol and sweetened with high-fructose corn syrup; try to avoid them. Mirin is great in marinades, dipping sauces, and Japanese-style soups and broths. If you don't have any, substitute a mixture of sake and sugar (about a tablespoon of sugar to a cup of sake).

MISO: A fermented soybean paste, miso is used as the basis of soups and sauces in Japanese cuisine. There are many types; recipes in this book specify red (aka) or white (shiro) miso. Miso keeps for a long time in the refrigerator.

MUSHROOMS: Fresh shiitake and oyster mushrooms are widely available. Avoid any that look dry or shriveled. Do not wash mushrooms; they already have a high water content. Brush them or wipe them with a dry towel if necessary. Store them in the refrigerator in waxed paper or in a paper bag, not plastic.

NORI: Nori is a processed form of seaweed widely used in Japanese cuisine as a wrapper for rice balls and sushi rolls and a garnish for soups and salads. Buy toasted nori sheets (or toast raw ones by waving them back and

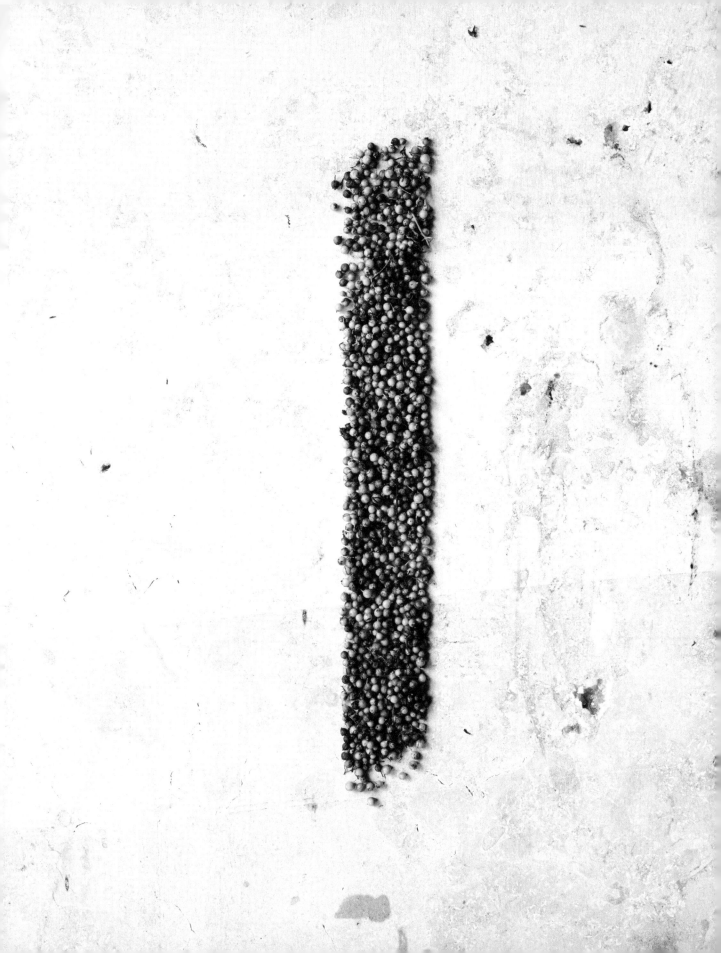

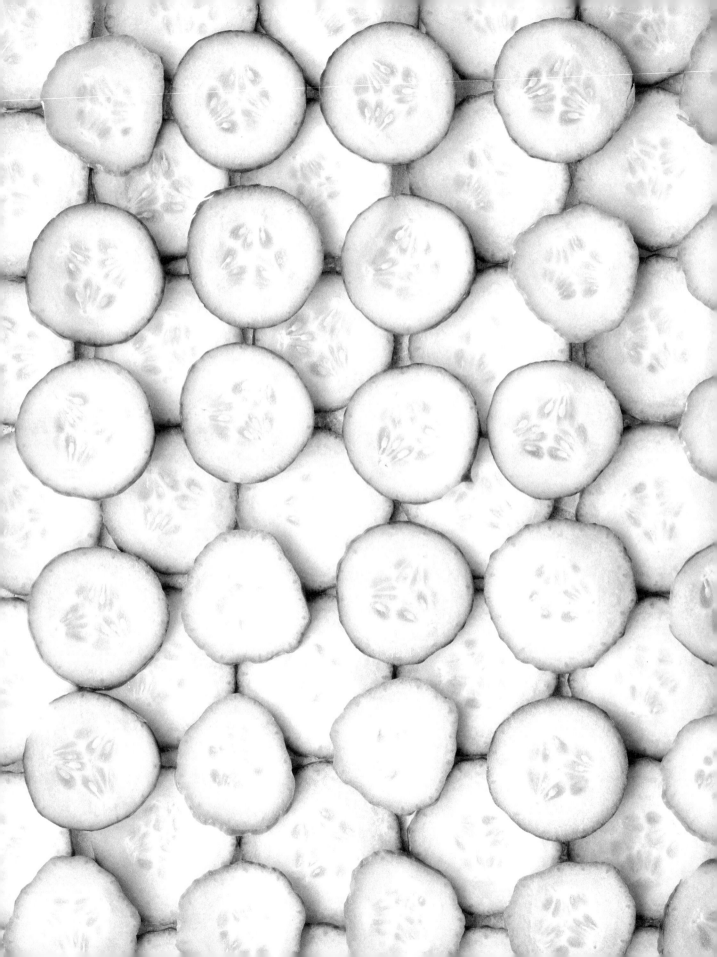

forth over a gas or electric burner for a minute or two until they turn green). You can buy flavored nori snacks and precut nori strips.

NUTS AND NUT MILK: Buy raw, whole nuts without any additives and store them in the refrigerator or freezer. Once nuts are roasted, they quickly go rancid, within a week or two if they are exposed to air, light, and heat. Make nut milk from raw cashews or blanched almonds by grinding them fine in a blender, then adding cold water and blending on high speed for several minutes. You can make nut milk rich or lean by varying the ratio of nuts to water; start with a 1 to 2 ratio. Store nut milk in a jar in the refrigerator for up to a week and shake well before using.

OLIVE OIL: Olive oil is the best general-purpose oil for sautéing, dressing salads and vegetables, and most cooking. Buy only extra-virgin olive oil, which has a rich flavor. And buy only oil that is packed in dark bottles or cans to prevent exposure to light, which hastens oxidation. Use it up quickly or store it in the refrigerator. (It will slowly congeal but you can easily liquefy it by placing the container in warm water.) Very good olive oils have a peppery "bite" or aftertaste, which comes from oleocanthal, a potent anti-inflammatory compound that is easily destroyed by exposure to air, light, or heat. Heat your pan first before adding olive oil to it.

PARMESAN CHEESE: Genuine Parmigiano-Reggiano cheese is a kitchen essential. Grate what you need on a Microplane grater and store the unused portion in plastic wrap in the refrigerator, where it will keep well. An acceptable, cheaper, but less flavorful substitute is grana Padano. Other good grating cheeses are aged Asiago, aged Gouda, and Swiss Sbrinz.

POULTRY: Because poultry—especially duck—is high in pro-inflammatory arachidonic acid (AA), it is used sparingly in the Anti-Inflammatory Diet. Turkey is a bit lower in AA than chicken. Buy organic, free-range poultry if possible to avoid residues of antibiotics and other chemicals added to conventional feed.

QUINOA: A quick-cooking, grainlike seed native to the high Andes of South America, quinoa is gluten-free with a higher protein content than many grains. Red and white varieties are available.

RICE-PAPER WRAPPERS: These thin, usually round sheets are used in Thai and Vietnamese cuisine to wrap various unfried rolls like fresh spring and summer rolls. They soften quickly in room-temperature water.

RICE VERMICELLI (NOODLES): Commonly used in Thai and Vietnamese cuisines, these gluten-free dried noodles come in a variety of thicknesses.

SAKE: Japanese rice wine. For cooking, inexpensive brands like Gekkeikan or Sho Chiku Bai will do; they are sold in many liquor stores and supermarkets. Refrigerate after opening.

SALT: Use a fine-grain sea salt with no additives.

SESAME OIL: Toasted sesame oil, often used as a garnish in Asian cuisine, is dark brown with a rich flavor. Store in the refrigerator.

SHALLOTS: More often used by professional chefs than home cooks, these onion relatives add great flavor to many dishes. Choose large, firm bulbs that do not appear dry or shrunken.

SHAOXING WINE: This is a traditional wine, originally from the Shaoxing region of eastern China, made from fermented rice. It is both a beverage and a cooking wine, available online and in Asian grocery stores. Dry sherry, such as a fino, is a good substitute.

SHICHIMI: Literally "seven spice," this is a ground mixture of various seeds and spices, including hot red pepper, roasted orange peel, hemp seeds, and nori. Shichimi is a great seasoning to keep on hand and is good sprinkled on soups, vegetables, fish, and more. See Basics (page 273) to make your own.

SHIITAKE: Shiitake are meaty, strong-flavored mushrooms commonly used in Chinese, Japanese, and Korean cooking. Soak dried shiitake in water to reconstitute them; cut off and discard the tough stems. Fresh shiitake are now widely available. Look for thick, firm ones with rounded caps; cut off and discard the stems before using them.

SICHUAN PEPPERCORNS: The dried outer husks of the tiny fruits of a tree native to China,

Sichuan peppercorns have a lemony flavor and a pronounced numbing effect on the tongue. They are readily available from Asian grocery stores, spice dealers, and online sites.

SMOKED PAPRIKA: Imported from Spain, this spice adds a rich, smoky flavor to soups, stews, beans, and other dishes. Store opened jars or cans in the refrigerator.

SOY SAUCE: A universal condiment in Asian cooking, soy sauce is known as *shōyu* in Japan. Look for naturally fermented brands with no additives that are low in sodium. If you are gluten-intolerant, use wheat-free brands. Store soy sauce in the refrigerator.

SPICES: You can buy an inexpensive electric spice grinder and grind whole spices as needed (see the next section for recommended brands). Most people like the convenience of ground spices, but they must be fresh. Once opened, they quickly go stale with exposure to air, light, or heat. Buy small containers of ground spices and store them in the refrigerator.

SRIRACHA SAUCE: A hot sauce made from ripe red chili peppers, vinegar, garlic, sugar, and salt, Sriracha is named for the coastal city of Si Racha in Thailand, where it may have originated. It has become very popular in North America and is easy to find in Asian sections of supermarkets as well as in specialty stores and online. Look for products without artificial color or preservatives, such as Shark brand from Thailand.

SUGAR: Small amounts of sugar are used as seasoning in some recipes in this book to balance salt and sour tastes. Unless otherwise specified, evaporated cane sugar is best. It is made from fresh sugarcane juice that is concentrated and crystallized and has a bit more color and flavor than white sugar. Muscovado sugar is an unrefined sugar that is used in place of brown sugar. It has a deep caramel flavor with notes of vanilla.

TAHINI: This sesame paste is ubiquitous in Middle Eastern cooking. Buy raw tahini, stir it well to mix in the separated oil, and store it in the refrigerator, where it will keep for a long time.

TEFF FLOUR: Teff is a tiny grain (the smallest in the world) native to the highlands of Ethiopia and Eritrea, where it is used to make a traditional spongy bread. Recently popular in North America because it is gluten-free, teff and teff flour are now available in natural-food stores and online from Bob's Red Mill (bobsredmill.com). Teff has a mild, nutty taste and is rich in minerals.

TOFU: Made from soy milk through a process similar to making cheese (heating, coagulating, separating liquid from and then pressing the curds), tofu is a high-quality vegetable-protein food eaten daily in Japan and China and now popular here. Buy organic brands. You will want firm or extra-firm varieties for most tofu recipes in this book. Drain off the packing liquid and replace with fresh water to store tofu that you don't use at once. Flavored, baked, pressed tofu comes dry-packed and refrigerated. It has a meaty texture and can be eaten as a snack right out of the package or used in many recipes in place of meat or poultry.

VEGETABLE BROTH: Cartons of good commercial vegetable broth, both with and without salt, are sold in natural-food stores and in supermarkets. Trader Joe's Organic Hearty Vegetable Broth is excellent.

VERMOUTH: Dry (white) vermouth is an herb-infused, fortified wine, much better for cooking than ordinary white wine. The best brands are imported from Italy and France. Store opened bottles at room temperature.

VINEGAR: Keep several types of vinegar in your pantry: red and white wine vinegars, sherry vinegar, rice vinegar (seasoned and unseasoned), and good balsamic vinegar. Many flavored vinegars are available; experiment with them.

WASABI: Often called Japanese horseradish, this pungent green condiment comes from the root of an aquatic plant cultivated mostly in Japan but now in North America too. It is often served with sushi and sashimi (raw fish). Commercial wasabi powder (to be mixed with cold water to the consistency of a paste) contains no actual wasabi; it is ordinary horseradish or mustard with green coloring added. You can find real wasabi products online (at realwasabi.com, for example) and in the refrigerated or frozen sections of some Asian groceries.

KITCHEN SUPPLIES

Having the right tools for the job makes cooking quick and enjoyable. The following are my go-to kitchen tools.

BLENDER: Blenders are convenient for making beverages, smoothies, and purees, but you may not need one if you have a food processor and a handheld immersion blender. The Vitamix is a versatile, high-performance blender that does much more than most, but it is quite expensive.

CITRUS JUICER: A sturdy manual juicer for lemons and limes is a kitchen necessity. Look for stainless-steel or coated-aluminum models. Norpro, Oxo, and Amco are good brands.

CITRUS ZESTER: You can remove the zest from oranges, lemons, and limes with a Microplane grater, or look for zesters made by Zyliss, Oxo, and Amco.

COOKWARE: Pots and pans generally come in six varieties: saucepans, sauté pans, stockpots, roasting pans, grill pans, and frying pans. Heavy-bottomed pots and pans are essential. I suggest stainless-steel 18/10 gauge with an aluminum core sealed between two layers of stainless steel; it conducts heat well and is suitable for all stovetops. By category:

- **SAUCEPANS:** There are usually five sizes, from 1-quart to 5½-quart.

- **SAUTÉ PANS:** Come in 8-, 10-, and 12-inch diameters. Slope-sided pans are easier to use.

- **STOCKPOTS:** 12-quart and up.

- **GRILL PAN:** One standard size. They're most effective on a gas stove (food may take longer to cook on electric stoves). Grill pans should be rubbed with oil before using.

Ceramic-coated nonstick cookware is a great innovation, making Teflon-coated pans obsolete. The best brand I have found is Scanpan CTX, made in Denmark and available in many models online. I use them all the time. Not only do they give excellent results, they are a snap to clean.

GARLIC PRESS: The best garlic presses are sturdy and push most of the garlic through the holes. Good brands are Zyliss Susi and Oxo.

GREEN STORAGE BAGS FOR PRODUCE: A new product, these reusable plastic bags supposedly work by absorbing and removing ethylene gas, a natural substance made by plants to accelerate ripening (and that eventually leads to spoilage). Many people find that the bags keep lettuce and other salad greens and vegetables fresher longer. Debbie Meyer Green Bags and Evert Fresh Green Bags are available online.

IMMERSION BLENDER: This is one of the great recent inventions for the home cook. The best product by far is the Swiss-made Bamix. Its powerful motor makes short work of pureeing soups right in the pots they are cooked in.

KNIFE SHARPENER: Get in the habit of sharpening your own knives regularly. The simplest and cheapest tools are handheld, pull-through, ceramic (not carbide) sharpeners. (Serious knife lovers disdain them, because they can strip off too much metal.) Electric knife sharpeners are a more expensive option and can take off even more metal; Smith's, Chef's Choice, and Wüsthof products are good. If your knives are very dull, take them to a professional for sharpening.

KNIVES: A set of good knives is a kitchen essential. You'll want an all-purpose chef's knife, a paring knife, and a serrated bread knife, at least. I also like a Japanese-style santoku knife for slicing and mincing.

Knives must be sharp—see entry on Knife Sharpener above.

MICROPLANE GRATER: Another wonderful recent invention, these rasp graters come in various sizes with holes suited to fine or coarse grating and zesting. Grated Parmesan is fluffier and more flavorful when prepared with a Microplane.

SPICE GRINDER: An electric spice grinder is a handy kitchen appliance for grinding whole spices as you need them for best flavor. KitchenAid, Krups, and Epica make good models.

TOASTER OVEN: A good toaster oven can bake and broil foods faster and cheaper than a regular oven. Breville's Smart Oven is outstanding.

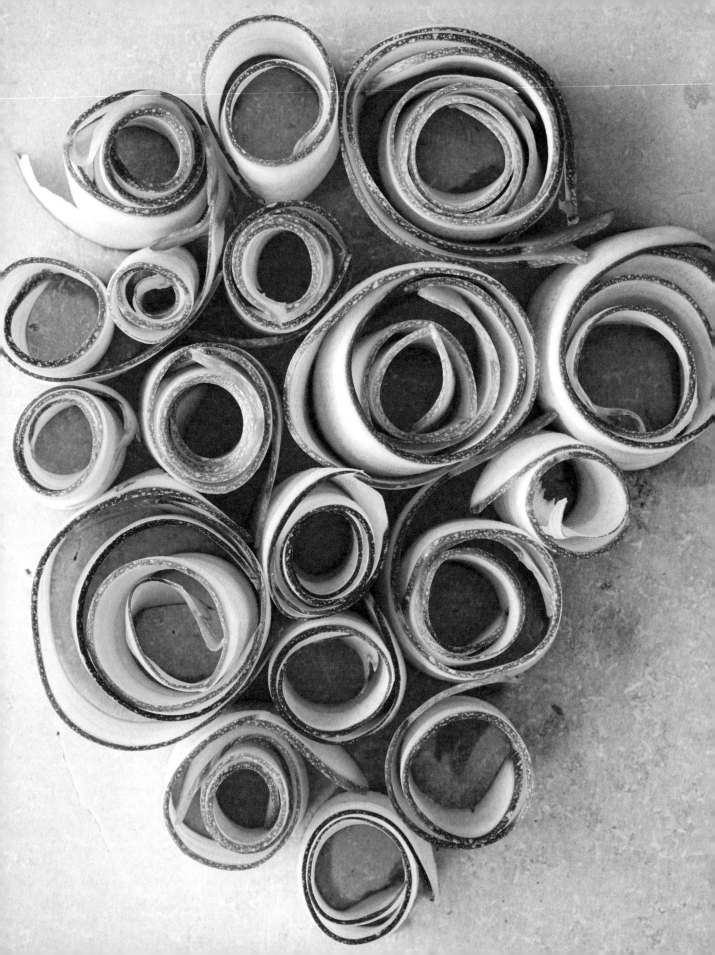

QUICK TIPS TO CREATE REAL FAST FOOD EVERY DAY

Organize your kitchen for efficiency. Everything needs a proper place so you can find it without searching.

- Put your everyday, most-used tools in the drawer closest to your work surface.

- Have your pantry essentials in the front of your cabinet.

- Keep a pinch bowl of sea salt on the counter along with a pepper mill.

- Move the tools you rarely use out of the way; they can go in a drawer across the room.

- Make sure your spices are visible and within easy reach.

- Organize your pots and pans. A couple of sauté pans, a soup pot, a small pot, and an eco-friendly nonstick are what you need to have front and center.

- Keep your knives sharp. When a knife is dull, you end up sawing through food. A sharp knife will cut your food in one stroke.

- Before you cook, clear the decks: Take everything you don't need off the counter.

- Read the recipe before you start cooking. Get a sense of the transitions involved from the preparation to the cooking and serving of the dish. A good understanding of a recipe allows you to improvise and stay several steps ahead to avoid any surprises.

- Consider preparing ingredients that need to be cleaned and chopped ahead of time; it's best to do it right when you bring them home from the market. Have all the ingredients for your dish out and ready to go. This will speed up your cooking time.

- Create a freezer inventory so you can have stocks, sauces, toasted nuts, and cooked dishes on hand in easy-to-use portion sizes. Label all of your containers with the date, contents, and quantity. When you're freezing food, always leave ½ to 1 inch of space at the top of the container to allow for expansion.

- Have the following on hand in the refrigerator: salad dressing, cooked grains, chopped vegetables, and cooked protein. Consider using the weekend to prepare these for the week.

- Create a recipe repertoire. Learn a few dishes well by cooking them over and over until you feel thoroughly familiar with them. You will be able to transfer what you learn to making other dishes.

- Pay attention to heat. If you cook in a pan that is too cold, your food will take longer to cook, lose moisture, and may not taste right. If your pan is too hot, you will burn your food.

- Clean as you go. Keep your work surface clear, and wash dishes and utensils as soon as you're done with them.

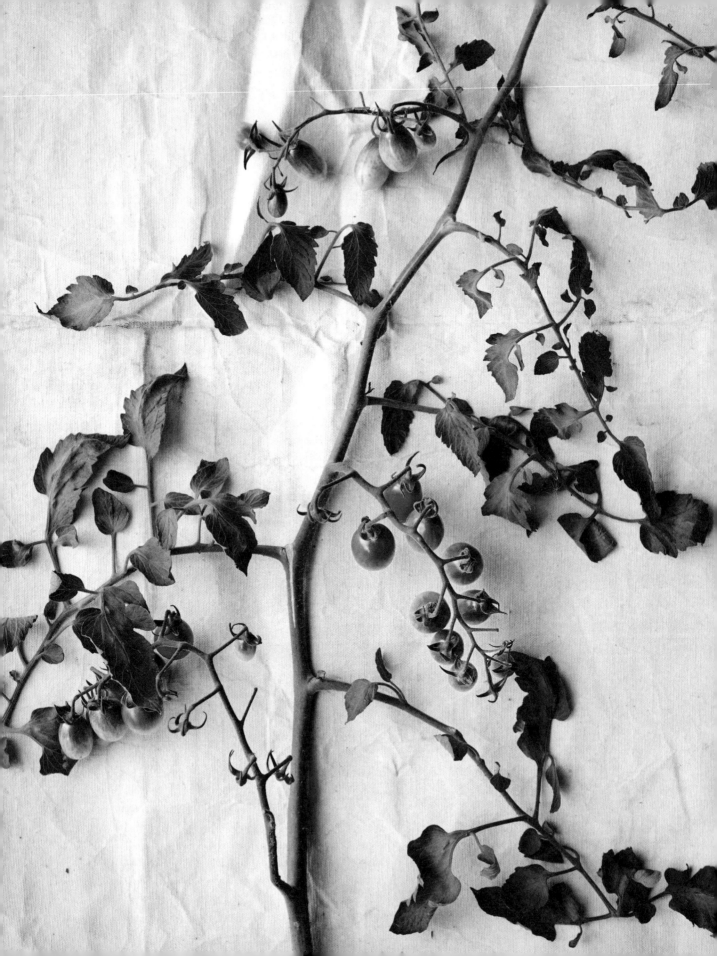

Starters

I've heard many people say they would be happy to have meals of nothing but appetizers and dessert. Really good starters may outshine main courses, although their intended functions are simply to wake up the senses, stimulate appetite, and create expectations of more substantial dishes to come. Starters should not be too filling, and, above all, they should be interesting. The recipes in this section follow these guidelines. They are diverse, easy, and fun to make and serve.

Recipes marked **veg** are vegetarian, those marked **v** are vegan, and those marked **gf** are gluten-free. The symbols **veg***, **v***, and **gf*** indicate recipes that can be modified to be vegetarian, vegan, or gluten-free by substituting or omitting specific ingredients.

BUFFALO MOZZARELLA BRUSCHETTA

SERVES 8, **VEG**

Bruschetta (pronounced "bruh-SKET-tah") is an Italian snack or appetizer of toasted bread rubbed with olive oil and seasonings and topped with various ingredients. The combination of garlic, tomatoes, and basil is classic; fresh mozzarella adds body. Buffalo mozzarella, made from the milk of the domesticated water buffalo, is a southern Italian delicacy, now widely available here packed in brine and refrigerated. The American product may not equal the Italian original, but it is still richer and creamier than cow's milk mozzarella, as well as higher in protein and calcium.

8 large slices country-style Italian bread

2 tablespoons extra-virgin olive oil

2 garlic cloves, pressed and allowed to sit for 10 minutes

3 tablespoons balsamic vinegar

¾ cup sliced fresh basil

1 cup halved cherry tomatoes

12 ounces buffalo mozzarella, torn into bite-size pieces

Sea salt and freshly ground black pepper, to taste

1. Brush the slices of bread liberally with olive oil and grill or toast until crisp and lightly browned.

2. Combine the remaining ingredients in a bowl and let sit for about 5 minutes so the flavors meld.

3. Taste and adjust the seasoning, adding more salt or pepper if needed. Spoon the mixture over the toasted bread and serve.

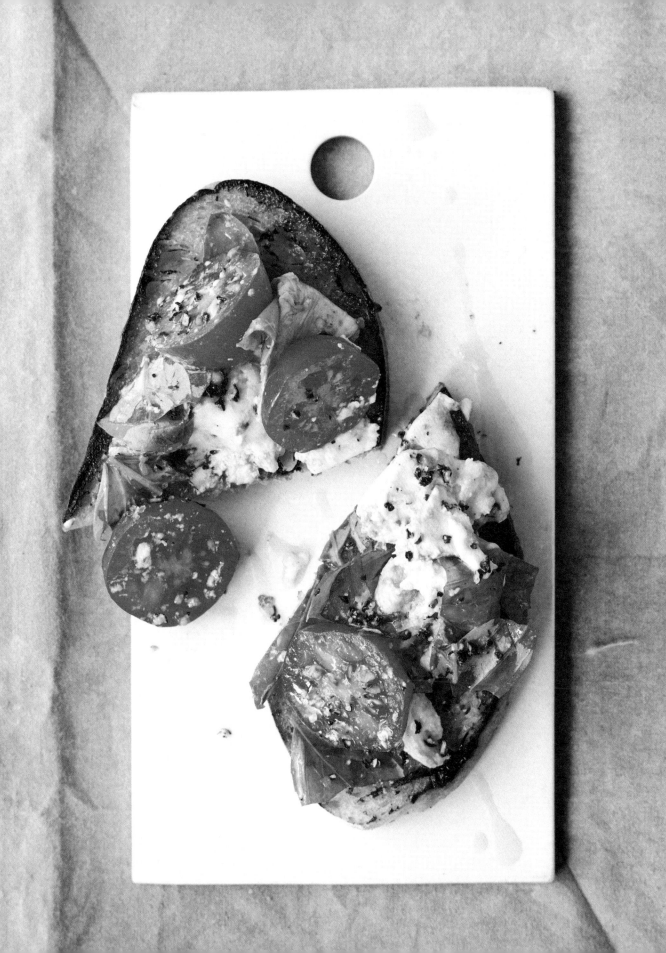

CHIPOTLE BLACK BEAN DIP

SERVES 6, **V, GF**

I've always preferred to cook with dried beans, but in the interest of quick preparation, I'm happy to say that several canned-bean varieties are quite acceptable, among them black beans. Add salt cautiously, because even after rinsing, canned beans may be salty. Chipotles are dried and smoked ripe jalapeño peppers. Their flavor is essential in this dip.

1 garlic clove, pressed and allowed to sit for 10 minutes

1 (15-ounce) can black beans, rinsed and drained

¼ cup roughly chopped white onion

¼ cup salsa (jarred or fresh)

2 tablespoons lime juice, or to taste

¼ cup fresh cilantro, leaves and tender stems, plus 2 tablespoons chopped fresh cilantro for garnish

¼ teaspoon chipotle chili powder, or more to taste

1 teaspoon ground cumin

½ teaspoon sea salt, or to taste

1 to 2 tablespoons water (optional)

1 small tomato, seeded and finely diced

1. Place all of the ingredients except the water, tomato, and chopped cilantro for garnish in the bowl of a food processor. Pulse until you reach a dip-like consistency.

2. If the mixture is too thick, continue to pulse, adding water by the tablespoon. Taste and adjust the seasoning with more salt or lime juice, if desired.

3. Transfer to a serving bowl, cover the dip, and place in the refrigerator to chill for at least 15 minutes. Garnish with diced tomatoes and chopped cilantro, and serve with vegetables or tortilla chips for dipping. The mixture can be stored in an airtight container in the refrigerator for up to 3 days.

FRESH MOZZARELLA and HEIRLOOM TOMATOES with KALE PISTACHIO PESTO with GARLIC SCAPES

SERVES 4, **VEG, GF**

Caprese salad with a twist. Fully ripe tomatoes in season are a must. If you do not wish to make the Kale Pistachio Pesto with Garlic Scapes, use regular basil pesto.

1½ pounds fresh mozzarella, at room temperature

3 large ripe heirloom tomatoes

⅔ cup Kale Pistachio Pesto with Garlic Scapes (page 270)

1. Slice the mozzarella and tomatoes into ½-inch-thick slabs. Place a slice of mozzarella on top of each tomato slice and arrange the stacks on a platter.

2. Put a dollop of pesto on each stack and serve.

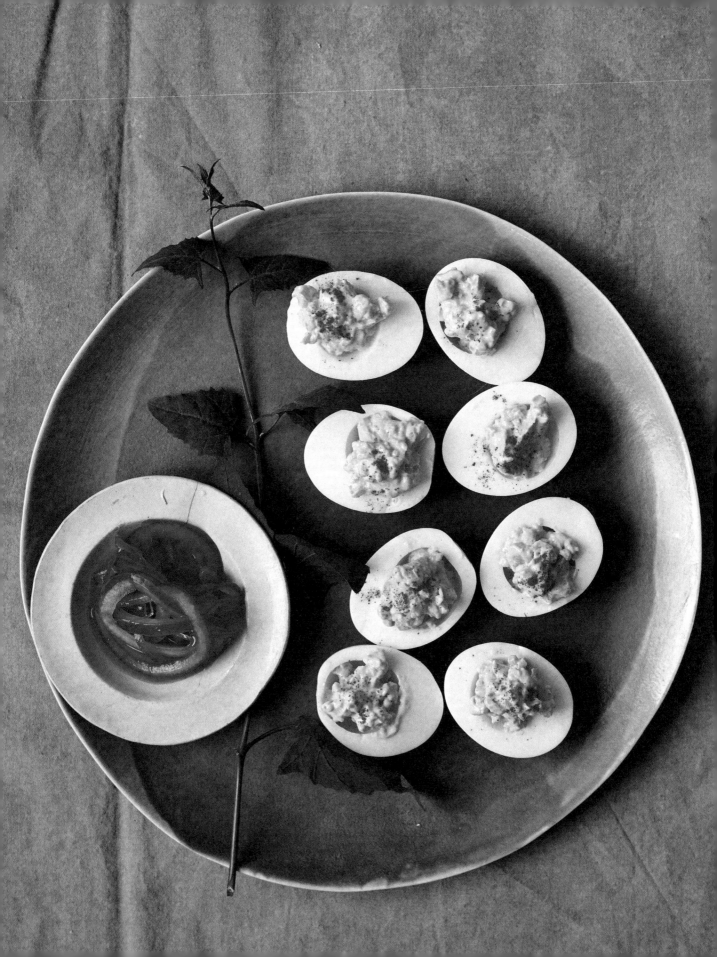

CURRY DEVILED EGGS

SERVES 4, **VEG, GF**

Deviled eggs are popular throughout Europe and have been for a long time. In the most common preparation, the yolks of hard-boiled eggs are mixed with mayonnaise and mustard and stuffed back into the halved whites with various garnishes. This version uses curry powder, lime juice, and a pinch of cayenne pepper to make them a bit more interesting, and the pickled-onion garnish is really special. A plate of cold deviled eggs is an attractive and tasty starter, especially in warm weather.

4 hard-boiled eggs, peeled

2 tablespoons mayonnaise

1½ teaspoons lime juice

¼ teaspoon curry powder

¼ teaspoon sea salt

2 pinches of cayenne pepper

Quick Pickled Onions (page 271)

1. Cut the eggs in half lengthwise. Put the yolks in a small bowl and set the whites on a plate.

2. Mash together the yolks with the mayonnaise, lime juice, curry powder, salt, and cayenne and mix until smooth.

3. Evenly disperse heaping teaspoons of the mixture into the egg-white cups. Garnish with a pickled onion or two.

GUACAMOLE

SERVES 4 TO 6, **VEG, V, GF**

What a shame to ruin this simple, traditional Mexican dish—with roots going back to the ancient Aztecs—by adding too many ingredients or ingredients that have no place in it (like mayonnaise and sour cream) or by reducing the avocado to a smooth puree. Great guacamole is chunky and rustic with just the right balance of salt, lime juice, onion, and chili. The buttery flesh of the Hass avocado, the one that has black, pebbly skin when ripe, is best. An avocado is ripe when it just yields to firm pressure from a thumb. Dark flesh indicates overripeness. Cut away any small dark spots, but discard the fruit if there is significant discoloration; the flesh will have an unpleasant off taste. Avocados are rich in healthy fat, perfectly consistent with the Anti-Inflammatory Diet. Slices of raw carrot, radish, celery, or cucumber make a satisfying alternative to chips. To prevent guacamole from darkening during storage, eat it all up!

4 large ripe avocados, preferably Hass

1 tablespoon lime juice, or more to taste

½ teaspoon sea salt

1 small red or white onion, finely chopped

¼ cup coarsely chopped fresh cilantro leaves

1 serrano chili, finely chopped (seeded for less heat)

1. Cut the avocados in half, remove the pits, and scoop the flesh out into a large bowl. Season with 1 tablespoon of the lime juice and the salt, and mash the flesh roughly with a fork.

2. Fold in the remaining ingredients. Taste and adjust with more salt and lime juice, if necessary. Serve with white, red, or blue tortilla chips or with sliced raw vegetables such as carrots, radishes, celery, or cucumber.

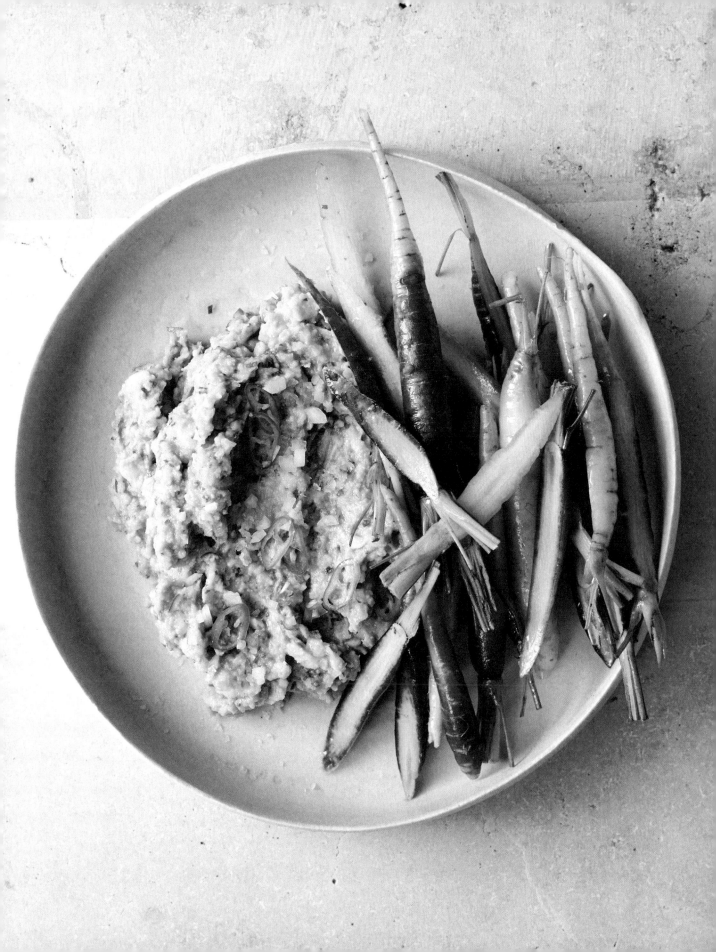

LEMONY HUMMUS with DUKKAH-SPICED PITA CHIPS

SERVES 6, **VEG, V, GF***

Most everybody likes hummus. The lemon juice and zest give this version an appealing freshness, and the mix of spices in the dukkah provides an exotic flair consistent with hummus's Middle Eastern origins. Try this for breakfast.

1 garlic clove, pressed and allowed to sit for 10 minutes

2 (15½-ounce) cans garbanzo beans, rinsed and drained

¼ cup lemon juice

2 teaspoons grated lemon zest

3 tablespoons raw sesame tahini

1½ teaspoons ground cumin

½ teaspoon plus a pinch of sea salt

Pinch of cayenne pepper

3 tablespoons plus 2 teaspoons extra-virgin olive oil

2 teaspoons Dukkah (page 273)

1 package whole-grain pita bread

1. Preheat the oven to 375°F and line a rimmed baking sheet with parchment paper.

2. Place the garlic, beans, lemon juice, lemon zest, tahini, cumin, ½ teaspoon of the salt, and cayenne into a food processor and blend until it is a smooth paste. With the food processor still running, add 2 tablespoons of the olive oil in a thin stream and blend until smooth and well combined. Transfer to a bowl, drizzle with 1 tablespoon of the olive oil, and sprinkle with 1 teaspoon of the Dukkah.

3. Meanwhile, cut the pita breads into quarters and split the layers. Arrange the quarters in a single layer on the baking sheet. Drizzle the bread with the remaining olive oil and salt. Bake 8 to 10 minutes or until crisp. Remove the chips from the oven and sprinkle with the remaining Dukkah.

4. Serve the hummus with the pita chips and your favorite raw vegetables. The hummus can be stored in an airtight container in the refrigerator for up to 5 days. The pita chips can be stored in an airtight container at room temperature for several days or frozen for later use.

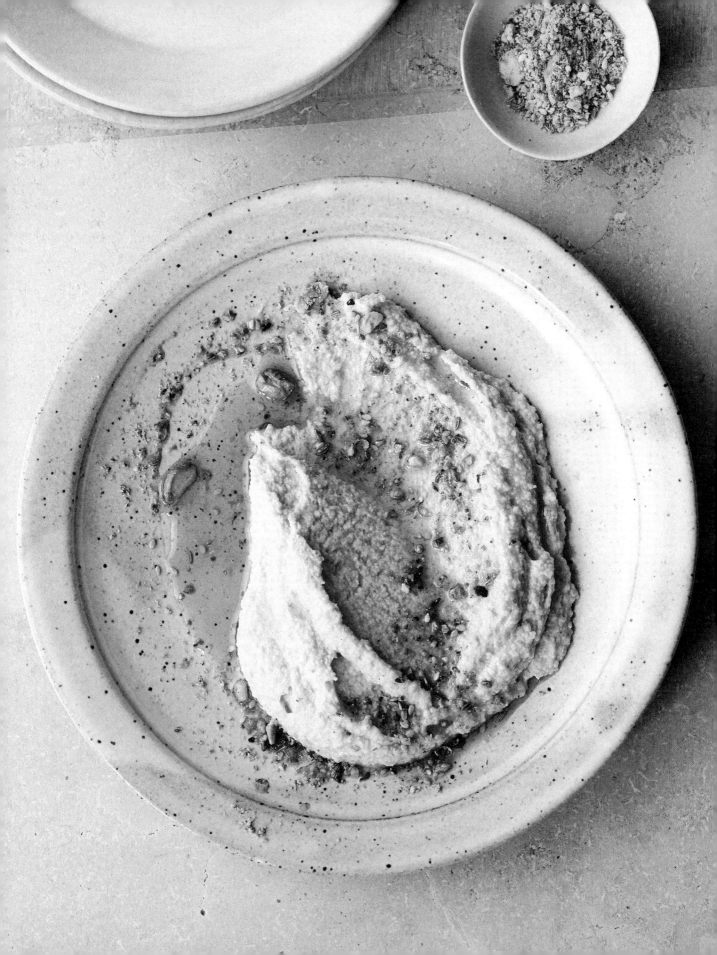

MISO TAHINI DIP

MAKES ¾ CUP, SERVES 6, **V, GF**

This is one of my favorite concoctions, very simple to prepare and versatile. I like to keep a container of it in my refrigerator. In addition to serving as a dip for raw vegetables, it is a savory spread that you can put on toasted bread, crackers, or wraps. You can also thin it with more water and drizzle it over steamed vegetables.

½ cup raw sesame tahini

1½ tablespoons red miso

¼ cup water (approximate)

2 garlic cloves, pressed and allowed to sit for 10 minutes

1. Mix the tahini and miso in a bowl until well combined. Add the water gradually while stirring. The mixture will first thicken and then turn smooth and creamy. Add just enough water to get the consistency you want for the dip. Add the pressed garlic and mix well.

2. Serve with vegetable crudités: carrot and celery sticks, cucumber spears, and red and orange bell pepper slices. Store leftovers in an airtight container in the refrigerator for up to a week.

ROQUEFORT CHEESE with HORSERADISH

SERVES 6, **VEG**

The pairing of blue cheese and horseradish might strike you as odd until you taste it. It is terrific. Use Prepared Fresh Horseradish if possible (page 268). It is a spectacular condiment that beats the commercial stuff hands down. Any blue-veined cheese will work here, but Roquefort, an ancient cheese made from sheep's milk, has a distinctive salty tang that marries well with the horseradish. Recent research has identified specific anti-inflammatory compounds in Roquefort that may have health benefits.

2 tablespoons Prepared Fresh
Horseradish (page 268)

Crackers

Celery stalks

½ pound Roquefort cheese,
at room temperature

Put about ½ teaspoon of the prepared horseradish on each cracker and celery stalk. Spread the cheese on top and serve.

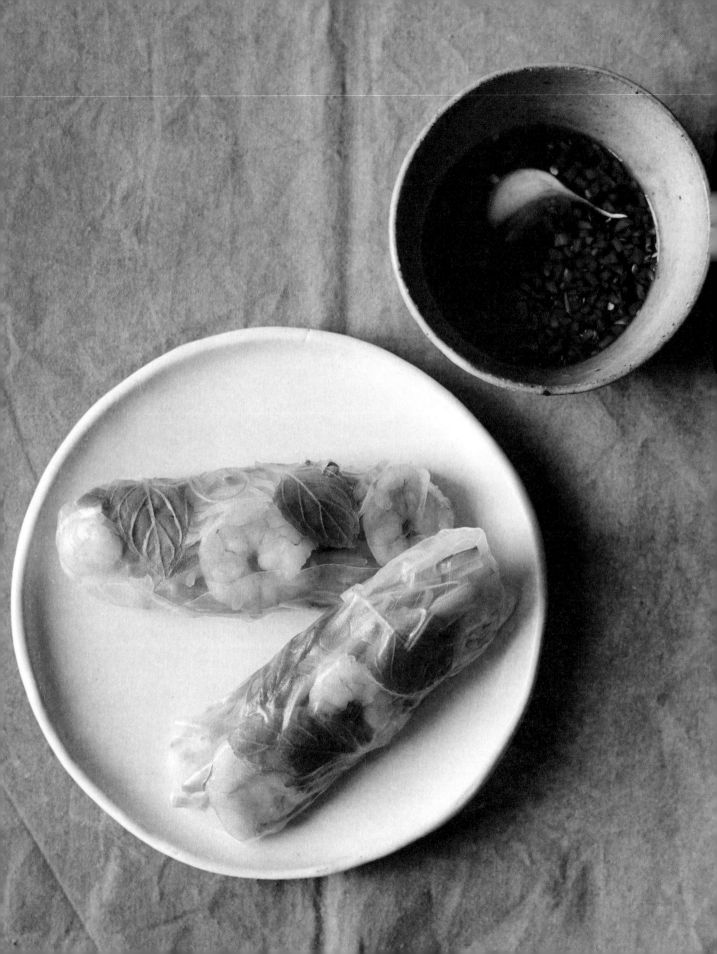

SHRIMP SUMMER ROLLS
with SPEARMINT and BASIL

SERVES 8, **GF**

These cold rice-paper rolls often appear as starters on menus at Vietnamese restaurants, along with vegan versions made with tofu (fresh or, better, baked and pressed). These light rolls with shredded vegetables and herbs are fresh and summery, and the slight chewiness of the rice-paper wrapper and rice vermicelli (both available online and from Asian grocery stores) provides a pleasant textural contrast to the vegetables and shrimp. A highly flavored dipping sauce (the Vietnamese call it *nuoc cham*) is a perfect complement.

DIPPING SAUCE

1 garlic clove, pressed and allowed to sit for 10 minutes

4 tablespoons lime juice

2 tablespoons plus 2 teaspoons evaporated cane sugar

3 tablespoons fish sauce

½ cup plus 2 tablespoons water

1 red chili, minced

ROLLS

8 ounces raw shrimp, peeled and deveined

2 ounces rice vermicelli

½ cup spearmint leaves

½ cup basil leaves

8 cilantro sprigs

1 small carrot, peeled and finely julienned

1 small English cucumber, finely julienned

2 scallions, white and light green parts only, halved and thinly sliced lengthwise

1 head Boston or green leaf lettuce, finely shredded

8 (8½-inch) rice-paper wrappers

1. Whisk the dipping sauce ingredients together, taste, and adjust the seasoning until the dressing is a nice balance of sweet, sour, salty, and spicy, and set aside.

2. Fill a saucepan with water and bring it to a boil. Reduce the heat to a simmer and add the shrimp. Gently cook for 1 to 1½ minutes or just until they are opaque and pink. Plunge the shrimp into a bowl of ice water to quickly cool. Drain the shrimp and slice them in half lengthwise.

3. Cook the rice noodles following the directions on the package. (You can use the shrimp water for this.) Rinse under cold running water, drain, and set them aside. Place the spearmint, basil, cilantro, carrot, cucumber, scallions, and lettuce in separate piles on a large platter; position the platter close to where you'll be rolling the summer rolls.

4. Fill a large bowl with hot tap water and completely submerge a sheet of rice paper for 20 seconds, until pliable. Transfer the sheet to a damp paper towel and add the fillings to the center of the wrapper. Start with three pieces of shrimp, laying them down cut-side up. Then add a small handful of rice noodles, a few spearmint and basil leaves, a sprig of cilantro, some cucumber, carrot, scallions, and lettuce.

5. Fold the bottom half of the wrapper up, covering the fillings, then fold in the sides. Press down firmly and roll up like a burrito. Transfer to a damp paper-towel-lined baking dish and cover with another damp paper towel. Repeat with the remaining rolls, then cover with plastic wrap. Serve chilled with the dipping sauce on the side.

SMOKED OYSTERS
with FRESH HORSERADISH

SERVES 6

Taste the horseradish to get a sense of its potency so that you do not put too much on these delicious appetizers. I like Wasa Sourdough Rye Crackers or other crispbread here. For the oysters, Crown Prince is my preferred brand.

1 can smoked oysters in pure olive oil (about 12 oysters)

12 rye crackers

2 tablespoons Prepared Fresh Horseradish (page 268), or to taste

1 tablespoon finely chopped fresh flat-leaf parsley leaves

1 lemon

Freshly ground black pepper (optional)

1. Drain as much oil as you can from the oysters and pat them dry, if necessary.

2. Spread the crackers with about ½ teaspoon of the prepared horseradish. Adjust the amount of horseradish to your taste. Place a smoked oyster on top of each cracker and top with a sprinkling of parsley, a squeeze of lemon, and freshly ground black pepper, if desired.

SIMPLEST SMOKED SALMON CANAPÉS

SERVES 8

Silky, rich cold-smoked salmon is an excellent source of protein and omega-3 fatty acids. Accented with crème fraîche or yogurt on small slices of whole-grain rye bread or crispbread and colorfully garnished with fresh dill or chives, it makes a delicious starter that couldn't be simpler to prepare. Good for breakfast as well.

4 slices dark whole-grain rye bread

½ cup crème fraîche or plain Greek yogurt

16 slices thinly sliced cold-smoked salmon

1 lemon

Dill sprigs or chopped chives

Freshly ground black pepper

1. Cut the rye bread into quarters.

2. Top each piece of bread with 1½ teaspoons crème fraîche or yogurt and 1 piece of smoked salmon. Squeeze a drop or two of fresh lemon juice on each canapé.

3. Garnish with a sprig of dill or chopped chives and a sprinkle of freshly ground black pepper.

NOTE: For a crispier canapé, toast the rye bread or use rye crispbread (like Wasa Sourdough Rye Crackers). If you want to get fancy, cut the smoked salmon slices into ribbons, then roll, twist, and place on top of the bread.

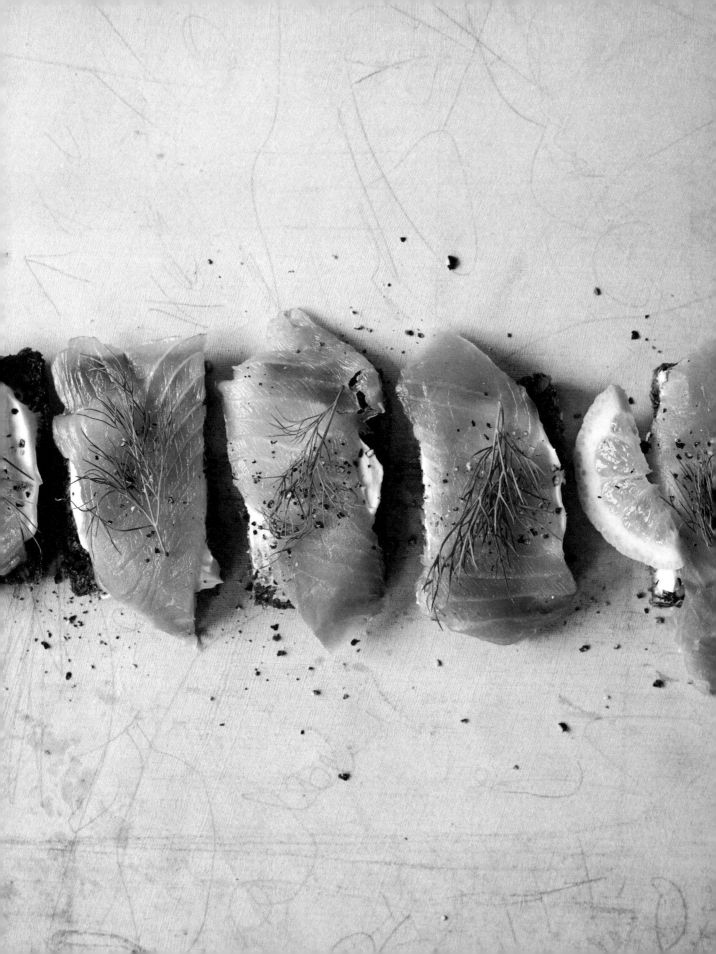

WALNUT-CRUSTED QUINCE
and MANCHEGO BITES

SERVES 12, **VEG**

Quince paste, known as *dulce de membrillo* in Spanish-speaking countries, is made by cooking the hard, tart flesh of this fruit (a relative of apples and pears) with water and sugar until it turns red and sticky and holds its shape. It's available in specialty grocery stores and online. In Spain, quince paste is commonly paired with manchego cheese, made from raw sheep's milk, as a breakfast item or snack. This recipe fancies up the combination with toasted spiced walnuts and chopped parsley and it also works as a breakfast dish.

1½ cups raw walnuts, toasted (page 274)

Pinch of sea salt

¼ teaspoon smoked paprika

1½ pounds quince paste, cubed

½ cup fresh flat-leaf parsley leaves

1½ pounds manchego cheese, cubed, at room temperature

1. Place the walnuts in a food processor and add a pinch of salt and the paprika. Pulse until the nuts are very finely chopped, then pour out onto a plate.

2. Roll and press each cube of quince paste in the walnuts until it is nicely coated. Thread onto a toothpick, place a leaf of parsley on top, and add a cube of manchego last. Thread the remaining quince paste, parsley, and cheese on toothpicks in the same way and serve.

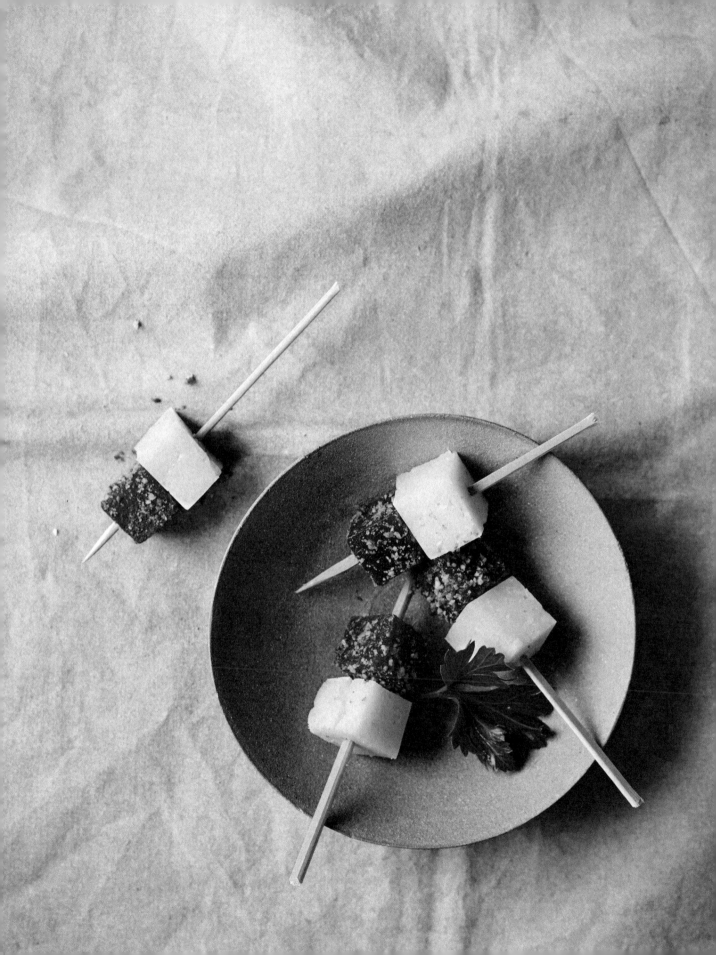

WARMED OLIVES
with CITRUS and HERBS

MAKES 1 CUP, SERVES 6, **V, GF**

This is super-quick and easy. The key is rinsing the olives well to get rid of the brine, then bathing them in lemon, olive oil, and herbs. Warming them greatly enhances their flavor. If you don't have access to Meyer lemons, use half a lemon and half an orange. This simple starter wows people every time. I like using Sicilian olive varieties—Cerignola and Castelvetrano.

1 cup assorted green and black olives, rinsed and drained

1 Meyer lemon, cut into quarters

1 tablespoon extra-virgin olive oil

2 garlic cloves, slivered

½ teaspoon fennel seeds

¼ teaspoon dried whole oregano

¼ teaspoon crushed red pepper flakes

1 sprig fresh rosemary

1. Put the olives in a bowl. Squeeze the juice from the lemon quarters over the olives, then add the lemon rinds, olive oil, garlic, fennel seeds, oregano, red pepper flakes, and rosemary. Stir until well combined.

2. Heat a skillet over medium heat. Add the olive mixture to the pan and sauté until the olives are heated through, about 4 minutes. Transfer the olives to a serving dish.

CURRIED SPICED MIXED NUTS

MAKES 2 CUPS, SERVES 8 TO 10, **V, GF**

These nuts are perfect as an appetizer with the previous recipe, Warmed Olives with Citrus and Herbs. As soon as you start to smell a wonderful aroma wafting from the oven, it's time to remove the nuts. They will continue to cook as they cool. You can easily double the recipe and freeze some for later use.

2 teaspoons extra-virgin olive oil

2 teaspoons grade B maple syrup

1 teaspoon curry powder

½ teaspoon sea salt

⅛ teaspoon cayenne pepper

½ cup raw walnuts

½ cup raw almonds

⅓ cup raw cashews

⅓ cup raw pistachios

1. Preheat the oven to 350°F and line a rimmed baking sheet with parchment paper.

2. In a medium bowl, whisk together the olive oil, maple syrup, curry powder, salt, and cayenne. Add the nuts and toss with a spatula until evenly coated. Spread the nuts evenly on the baking sheet.

3. Bake for 10 to 12 minutes and stir them about halfway through. Nuts are done when they are aromatic and slightly golden. Let them cool to room temperature, then use a metal spatula to loosen them from the parchment. Transfer to a serving dish or an airtight container. Store in the freezer for up to a month.

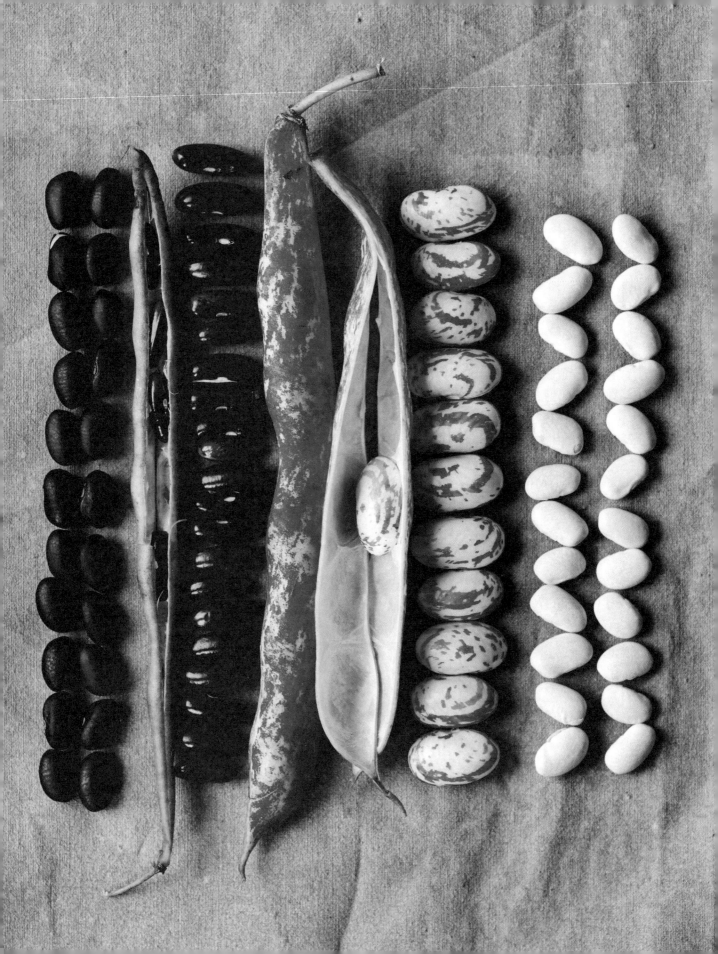

Soups

Thin or thick, hot or cold, simple or complex, soups are loved by most people and give the home cook opportunities to be creative with ingredients that are in season and on hand. You can make soups in quantity and serve them over several days or freeze them for later use. Light soups make good first courses; more robust ones can be meals in themselves, perhaps with a salad. In this section you'll find a wide variety of soups, some inspired by Asian cuisines, others taken from the culinary traditions of Mexico or Italy. Like other recipes in this book, all are quick and easy to make once you assemble the ingredients and do the usual slicing and chopping.

Recipes marked **veg** are vegetarian, those marked **v** are vegan, and those marked **gf** are gluten-free. The symbols **veg***, **v***, and **gf*** indicate recipes that can be modified to be vegetarian, vegan, or gluten-free by substituting or omitting specific ingredients.

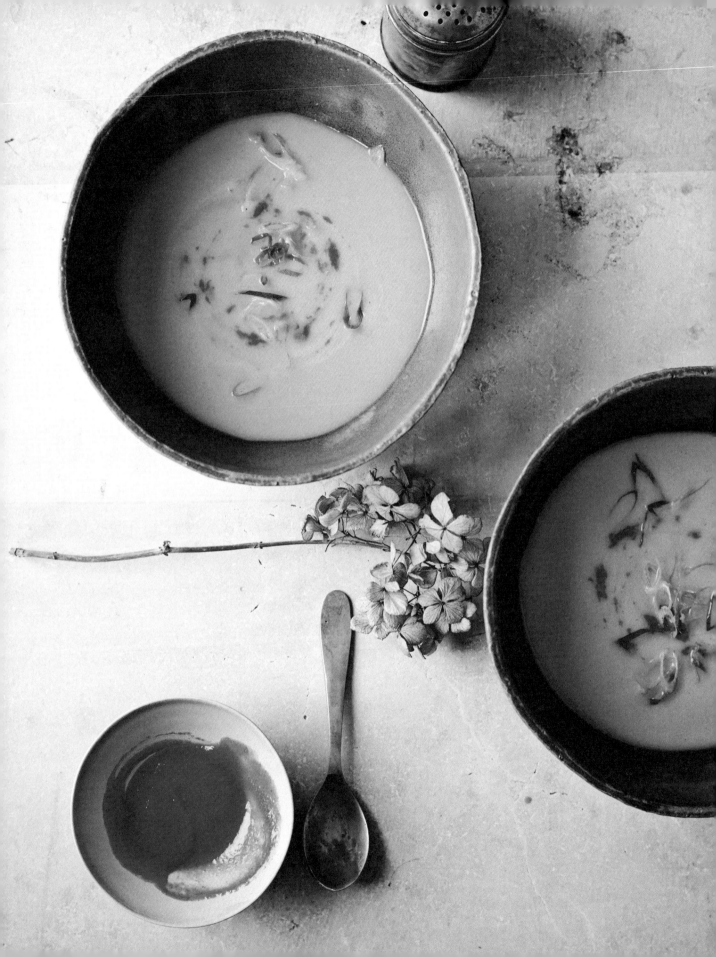

FIVE-SPICE WINTER SQUASH SOUP

SERVES 4 TO 6, **V**, **GF**

Chinese five-spice powder is a prepared mixture of ground spices, most commonly star anise, cinnamon, cloves, toasted fennel seeds, and toasted Sichuan peppercorns. Some versions add ginger, nutmeg, or orange peel or use black peppercorns in place of the Sichuan variety. In Chinese restaurants, five-spice powder is mostly used in rubs for meats and seafood. It also adds warm flavor notes to marinades and sauces. Here, a mere ½ teaspoon of the powder gives distinctive depth of character to this nutrient-rich soup with the subtle sweetness of butternut squash, pear, and a touch of maple syrup.

1 tablespoon grapeseed oil

1 pound butternut squash, peeled, seeded, and cut into ½-inch pieces

1 Asian (or russet) pear, peeled, cored, and roughly chopped

3 large shallots, chopped

2 garlic cloves, pressed and allowed to sit for 10 minutes

4 scallions, finely sliced (keep white and light green parts separate)

1 tablespoon dry sherry

2 teaspoons grade B maple syrup

½ teaspoon Chinese five-spice powder

Sea salt and freshly ground black pepper, to taste

4 cups Quick Vegetable Stock (page 266) or store-bought vegetable broth

Sriracha or other hot sauce

1. Heat the oil in a soup pot over medium-high heat. Add the squash and sauté until golden, about 6 minutes.

2. Add the pear, shallots, garlic, and white parts of the scallions and continue cooking until the shallots are translucent, about 2 minutes.

3. Stir in the sherry, maple syrup, five-spice powder, salt, and pepper and cook for a minute or two. Add the broth, raise the heat to high, and bring the soup to a boil. Reduce the heat to medium-low, partially cover the pot, and cook at a low boil for 8 to 10 minutes or until the squash is tender.

4. Puree the soup in a blender or with an immersion blender. Taste and adjust with salt or maple syrup, if necessary. Serve garnished with the green parts of the scallions and a dash of Sriracha sauce, to taste.

BEET and CARROT BORSCHT

SERVES 4 TO 6, **VEG, V*, GF**

Borscht, which has its roots in Russian and Eastern European cuisines, is traditionally made with shredded beets and cabbage in beef broth. This chunky vegetarian take is full of flavor surprises, including the anti-inflammatory spices cumin, coriander, and caraway.

3 tablespoons extra-virgin olive oil

2 medium onions, diced

¾ teaspoon plus a pinch of sea salt

1 teaspoon ground cumin

1 teaspoon ground coriander

1 teaspoon caraway seeds

Pinch of crushed red pepper flakes

3 beets, peeled and cut into ½-inch dice

2 large carrots, peeled and cut into ½-inch dice

6 cups Quick Vegetable Stock (page 266) or store-bought vegetable broth

1 tablespoon lemon juice

6 teaspoons plain yogurt

¼ cup chopped fresh dill

1. Heat the olive oil in a soup pot over medium heat, then add the onions and a pinch of salt. Sauté until the onions start to turn golden, about 4 minutes. Stir in the cumin, coriander, caraway, and red pepper flakes and sauté until well combined.

2. Add the beets and carrots and another ¼ teaspoon of salt, then stir and cook for about a minute. Add the broth and the remaining salt. Bring to a boil, then reduce the heat to medium, cover, and simmer until the beets and carrots are tender, about 20 to 25 minutes. Add the lemon juice, and adjust the seasoning, if necessary.

3. To serve, garnish each bowl with a teaspoon of yogurt and a sprinkle of dill.

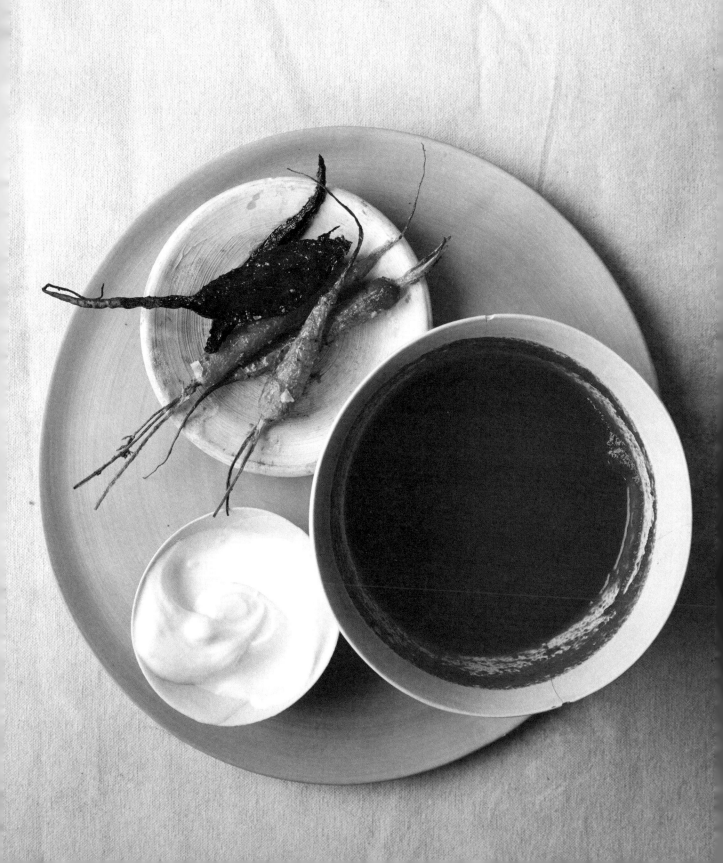

SPRING GREEN SOUP

SERVES 4, **VEG**, **V***, **GF**

This brightly colored soup is delicate but flavorful and a snap to make. It's good both warm and chilled. For a vegan version, use Cashew Milk (see page 275) instead of yogurt.

2 tablespoons extra-virgin olive oil

1 leek, white and light green parts only, thinly sliced

1 teaspoon sea salt

3 cups Quick Vegetable Stock (page 266) or store-bought vegetable broth

2 cups or ½ bag (about 4½ ounces) tightly packed baby spinach or prepacked spinach

2 cups (10 ounces) frozen green peas, thawed

1 cup plain Greek yogurt, crème fraîche, or cashew milk

¼ cup chopped fresh flat-leaf parsley leaves

1 tablespoon coarsely chopped fresh spearmint

1 teaspoon lemon juice

1 tablespoon chopped fresh chives

1. Heat the oil in a soup pot over medium heat, add the leeks and ¼ teaspoon of salt, and sauté for 3 to 4 minutes until just tender and wilted. Add the broth and bring to a slow boil. Turn off the heat and stir in the spinach and peas.

2. Carefully transfer the hot soup to a blender. (Or, better, use an immersion blender right in the pot.) Add the yogurt, parsley, spearmint, remaining salt, and lemon juice. Blend on high speed until the soup is very smooth.

3. To serve, garnish each bowl with chopped chives. Serve warm, at room temperature, or cold.

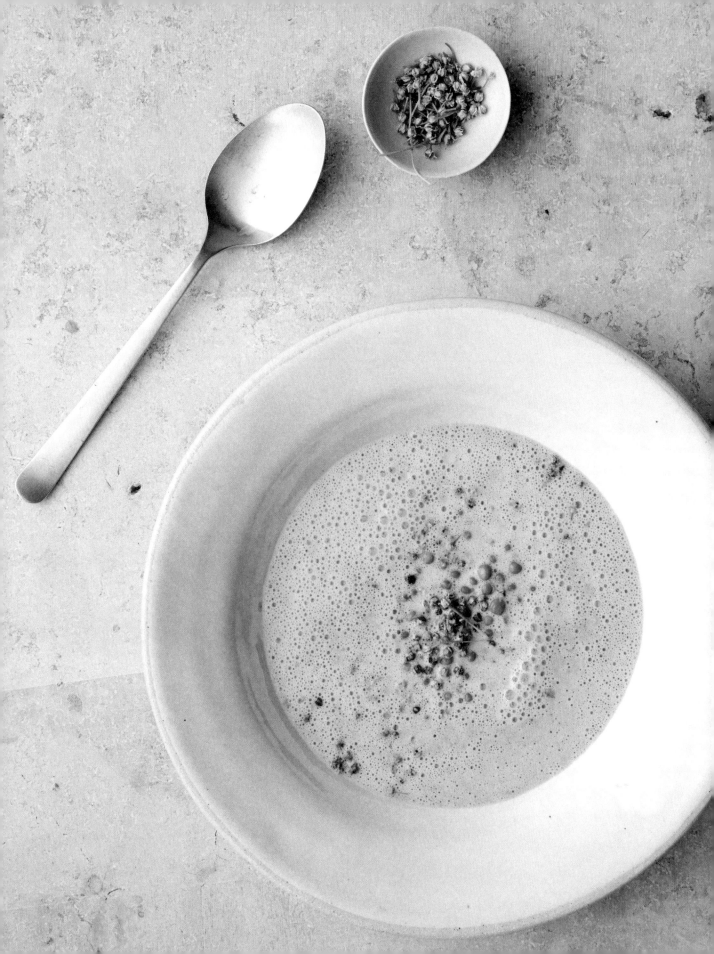

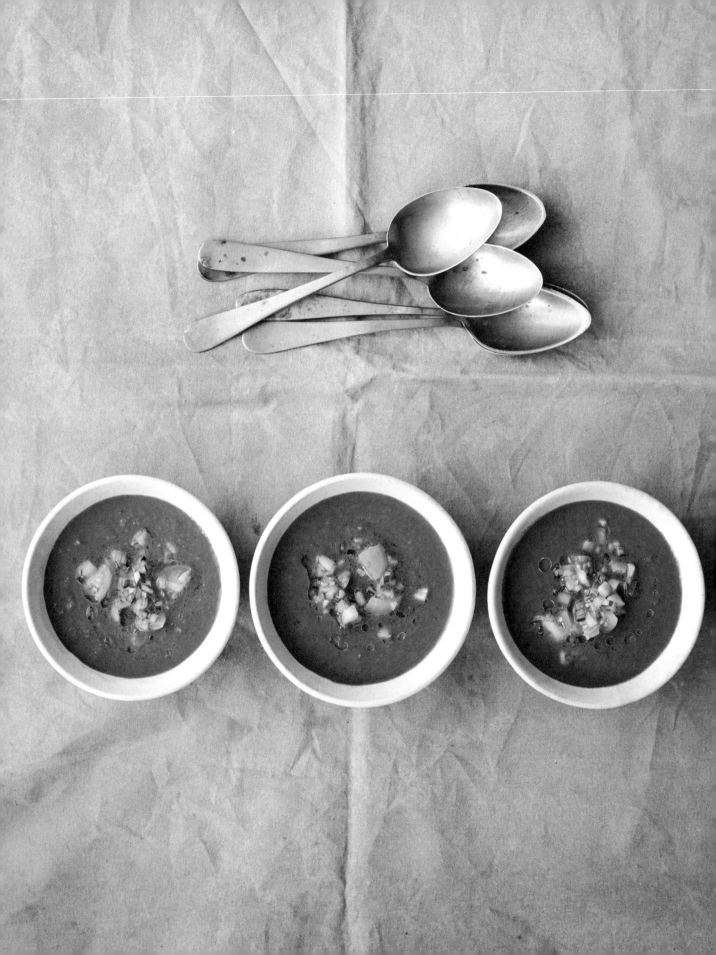

KALE and GREEN OLIVE GAZPACHO

SERVES 4, **V**, **GF***

A novel take on gazpacho using kale instead of tomatoes is the base for this super-quick and tasty chilled soup that's loaded with nutrients. Giving the kale a brief dunk in boiling water takes away any bitterness of the raw leaves. Salsa and croutons make this soup even more special.

6 cups stemmed roughly chopped black (lacinato) kale (about 2 bunches)

1 garlic clove, pressed and allowed to sit for 10 minutes

¼ cup extra-virgin olive oil, plus more for finishing

1 tablespoon plus 1 teaspoon lemon juice

1 cucumber, peeled, seeded, and cut into chunks

½ cup loosely packed fresh basil leaves

½ cup (about 20) halved, pitted green olives, rinsed

¼ cup loosely packed fresh flat-leaf parsley leaves

⅛ teaspoon crushed red pepper flakes

½ teaspoon sea salt

SALSA FRESCA

¼ cup finely diced red onion

¼ cup diced small cucumber, peeled and seeded

1 small jalapeño, seeded and diced

8 to 10 cherry tomatoes, quartered

1 tablespoon minced fresh basil

1 tablespoon extra-virgin olive oil

2 teaspoons lemon juice

¼ teaspoon sea salt

½ cup homemade croutons (page 274) (optional)

1. Bring a large pot of salted water to a boil over high heat. Plunge the kale in the boiling water and push it down with tongs for 30 to 60 seconds, until it turns a bright emerald green. Drain the kale in a colander and rinse well with cold water. Put the wet kale (do not squeeze it), 2 cups of water, and the remaining soup ingredients into a blender and blend on high for 1 minute or until the soup is completely smooth.

2. Transfer the soup to a lidded container and chill for two hours. Check for seasoning; you may want to add another pinch of salt or a squeeze of lemon.

3. Toss together all the Salsa Fresca ingredients except the croutons. To serve, garnish each bowl of soup with a tablespoon or two of the Salsa Fresca and a drizzle of olive oil. Add croutons, if desired, at the last second.

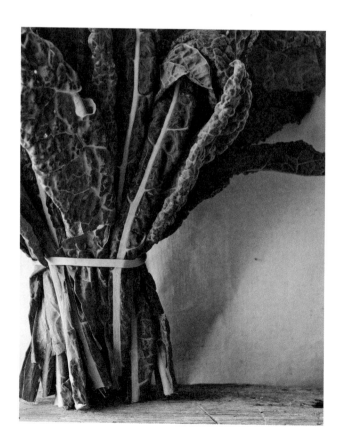

Fast Food, Good Food

BROCCOLI and PARMESAN SOUP

SERVES 4, VEG*, V*, GF

A very simple, quick soup consisting of broccoli briefly cooked in seasoned broth, then pureed right in the pot with an immersion blender. Chopped basil and a good quantity of freshly grated Parmesan cheese add flavor and richness. If you serve this soup with grilled or toasted bread, it makes a light meal.

3 tablespoons extra-virgin olive oil

3 garlic cloves, pressed and allowed to sit for 10 minutes

¼ teaspoon crushed red pepper flakes, or more to taste

2 pounds broccoli, trimmed and cut into small florets, stalks peeled (to remove fibrous outer layer) and cut into chunks

Sea salt, to taste

4 cups Quick Vegetable Stock (page 266) or store-bought vegetable or chicken broth

¼ teaspoon freshly ground nutmeg, or more to taste

¼ cup finely chopped fresh basil leaves

1 cup grated Parmesan cheese, or more to taste

1. Heat the oil in a soup pot over low heat. Add the garlic and red pepper flakes, and let infuse into the oil for 3 minutes.

2. Raise the heat to medium-high, add the broccoli florets and stalks, and season with salt. Sauté the broccoli for a couple of minutes, then pour in one cup of the broth. Reduce the heat to medium-low, cover the pot, and let the broccoli steam for 3 to 4 minutes until just tender. Add more broth during the cooking process if needed to prevent the pot from going dry.

3. Pour in the remaining stock and bring the soup to a simmer. Add the nutmeg and basil and blend the soup directly in the pot with an immersion blender until very smooth.

4. Shut off the heat and stir in the grated cheese. Taste and adjust with more Parmesan, salt, or red pepper flakes, if needed.

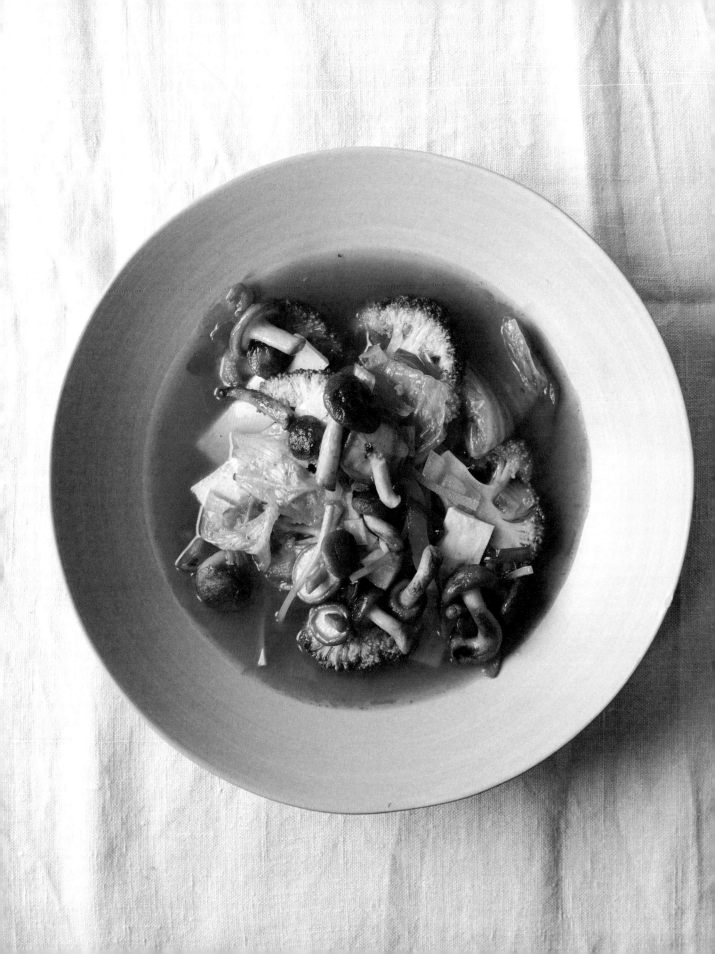

KOREAN KIMCHI SOUP
with TOFU and VEGETABLES

SERVES 6, **VEG***, **V***, **GF**

Fermented cabbage in soup? Germans, Poles, and other Eastern European peoples make soup from sauerkraut, often with sausages and vegetables. Koreans do the same with their beloved kimchi, fermented Napa cabbage strongly flavored with ginger, scallion, garlic, and hot red pepper. Despite the Koreans' love of meat, they enjoy vegetarian versions like this one made with shiitake mushrooms and baked pressed tofu. Although easy to prepare, this is a complex soup, filling and satisfying. You can add more protein and turn this into a one-dish meal by adding raw, peeled shrimp to the soup when you put in the broccoli.

1 tablespoon grapeseed oil

2 teaspoons toasted sesame oil

1 large yellow onion, diced

8 ounces shiitake or button mushrooms, thinly sliced

2 teaspoons peeled, grated ginger

2 teaspoons crushed red pepper flakes

4 garlic cloves, pressed and allowed to sit for 10 minutes

1 cup kimchi, drained, ¼ cup juice, or more to taste, reserved

5½ cups Quick Vegetable Stock (page 266) or store-bought vegetable or chicken broth

2 packages baked pressed tofu, cut into 1-inch chunks

2 carrots, peeled and julienned

1 red bell pepper, seeded and thinly sliced

1 tablespoon evaporated cane sugar, or more to taste

1 tablespoon low-sodium soy sauce, or more to taste

2 cups broccoli florets

6 scallions, white and light green parts only, finely sliced

1. Heat the grapeseed and sesame oil in a soup pot over medium-high heat. Add the onion and sauté for 2 minutes. Add the mushrooms, ginger, and red pepper flakes and continue to cook while stirring for 3 minutes.

2. Add the garlic and kimchi and stir-fry for 3 minutes more, until the garlic is aromatic. Add the broth, tofu, carrots, bell pepper, reserved kimchi juice, sugar, and soy sauce and simmer, partially covered, for 6 to 8 minutes.

3. Add the broccoli and cook for 2 minutes until just tender and crisp. Adjust the seasoning with more sugar, soy sauce, red pepper flakes, or kimchi juice to taste. Remove from the heat. To serve, garnish each bowl with scallions.

QUICK BLACK BEAN SOUP

SERVES 6, **VEG*, V*, GF**

Using canned black beans is a big time-saver in making this filling soup, which gets its richness from a balanced array of spices rather than fat. Chipotle peppers are dried, ripe, smoked jalapeños, sold whole, ground, or canned in a thick, spicy tomato sauce (adobo). It is the canned variety, along with its sauce, that really enlivens this soup. Go easy on the salt until the end, because both the beans and the adobo sauce may be salty. The garnishes of avocado, cilantro, scallion, and lime are essential.

2 tablespoons extra-virgin olive oil

1 large yellow onion, chopped

1 teaspoon ground allspice

2 teaspoons ground cumin

1½ teaspoons dried oregano

2 Turkish bay leaves or ⅔ of a California bay leaf

Sea salt, to taste

4 garlic cloves, pressed and allowed to sit for 10 minutes

1 jalapeño pepper, seeded and finely diced

1 canned chipotle pepper in adobo, seeded and finely chopped

1½ tablespoons adobo sauce from can, or more to taste

3 cups Quick Vegetable Stock (page 266) or store-bought vegetable or chicken broth

2 (15-ounce) cans black beans, rinsed and drained

1 cup fire-roasted tomatoes or diced tomatoes, drained

2 tablespoons lime juice

2 avocados, diced

2 scallions, finely sliced

¼ cup chopped fresh cilantro leaves

Lime wedges

1. Heat the oil in a large soup pot over medium-high heat. Sauté the onion for 6 to 8 minutes or until soft and beginning to brown. Add the allspice, cumin, oregano, and bay leaves, and season the onions lightly with salt.

2. Reduce the heat to medium and add the garlic, jalapeño, chipotle, and adobo sauce. Cook for 2 minutes while stirring, until the garlic is aromatic and the chilies have softened.

3. Add the broth, beans, tomatoes, and lime juice; stir to combine. Cover the pot and simmer the soup for 6 to 8 minutes to let the flavors come together.

Discard the bay leaves and partially blend the soup in the pot with an immersion blender. Remove from the heat. Taste and adjust with more salt or adobo sauce, if needed.

4. Serve each bowl garnished with a few pieces of avocado, scallions, cilantro, and a wedge of lime.

QUICK CORN CHOWDER

SERVES 6, **V, GF**

An iconic summer soup, corn chowder is too often overly rich with bacon and quantities of butter, cream, or half-and-half, plus the added glycemic load of potatoes. This version uses olive oil and a moderate amount of cashew milk. Of course, fresh corn kernels, cut from the cob, are one of summer's treats, but the new frozen supersweet corn now widely available allows you to enjoy this soup throughout the year with minimal preparation time. Smoked paprika, a pantry essential, adds greatly to the flavor.

2 tablespoons extra-virgin olive oil

1 onion, sliced

1 pound frozen supersweet yellow or white corn

3 cups Quick Vegetable Stock (page 266) or store-bought vegetable broth

1 cup Cashew Milk (page 275)

1 teaspoon smoked paprika, or more to taste

Sea salt and freshly ground black pepper, to taste

6 tablespoons chopped fresh chives or chive-infused olive oil

1. Heat the olive oil in a soup pot over medium-high heat. Add the onions and sauté, stirring occasionally, until they are translucent and beginning to color, about 5 minutes. Add the frozen corn and stir to mix well. Add the vegetable broth, raise the heat to high, and bring to a boil.

2. Cover the pot, lower the heat, and boil gently for 5 minutes. Add the Cashew Milk, smoked paprika, salt, and pepper, and continue to cook for another minute.

3. Remove the pot from the heat and use an immersion blender to puree the soup. (You can do this in a regular blender, but let the soup cool first to avoid splashing hot liquid.)

4. Heat the pureed chowder over low heat to desired serving temperature. Adjust the seasoning if necessary. To serve, top each bowl with a tablespoon of chopped chives or a swirl of chive-infused oil.

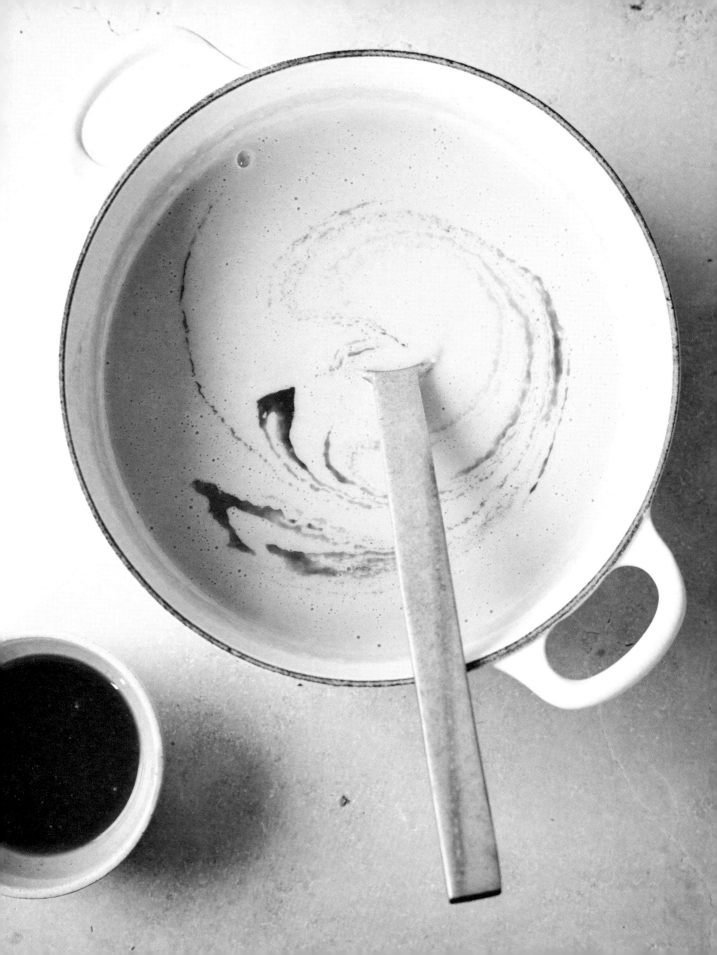

QUICK RED LENTIL DAL

SERVES 6, **V, GF**

This is a quick version of the lentil dal that is a staple of Indian cuisine. It's full of anti-inflammatory spices. Lentils are a good source of vegetable protein, and their slow-digesting carbohydrates and fiber help stabilize blood sugar.

2 tablespoons extra-virgin olive oil

1 onion, finely diced

½ teaspoon plus a pinch sea salt

1 tablespoon peeled, minced fresh ginger

1 teaspoon curry powder

½ teaspoon ground cumin

½ teaspoon ground coriander

¼ teaspoon ground cinnamon

1 (14.5-ounce) can diced tomatoes, drained, juice reserved

8 cups Quick Vegetable Stock (page 266) or store-bought vegetable broth

2 cups dried red lentils, rinsed well

1 teaspoon lime juice

2 tablespoons finely chopped fresh cilantro

1. Heat the olive oil in a soup pot over medium heat. Add the onion and a pinch of salt and sauté until translucent, about 4 minutes. Add the ginger, curry powder, ground cumin, coriander, cinnamon, and a pinch of salt and sauté for about 3 minutes more.

2. Add the drained tomatoes and ¼ teaspoon of the salt and sauté for 2 minutes. Pour in ½ cup of the broth and the reserved juice from the tomatoes to deglaze the pot, stirring to loosen any bits stuck to the bottom. Cook until the liquid is reduced by half, about 5 minutes. Add the lentils and stir well, then add the remaining broth. Increase the heat to high and bring to a boil. Decrease the heat to low, cover, and simmer until the lentils are tender, about 20 minutes.

3. Stir in the remaining salt and simmer for 5 minutes. Stir in the lime juice and serve each bowl garnished with cilantro.

SHIRO MISO SOUP

SERVES 4, **V**, **GF**

This simple soup is Japanese comfort food, good for everything from a cold to fatigue to an overworked digestive system. Miso is a traditional fermented food, made for centuries in Japan, with myriad health benefits. To avoid damaging the beneficial microorganisms it contains, never cook it. Shiro (white) miso is made from salted barley, rice, and soybeans inoculated with a fungus (*Aspergillus oryzae*) cultivated on rice that is also used to make sake and soy sauce. The flavor of shiro miso is milder and sweeter than darker types made with more soybeans. All miso is salty and needs to be diluted with water or other ingredients until the salt level is right for you. This quick and easy recipe is one of my favorite soups. I even like it for breakfast.

2 teaspoons grapeseed oil

½ teaspoon toasted sesame oil

1 onion, thinly sliced

1 large carrot, peeled, sliced into thin half-moons

3 (¼-inch) slices unpeeled ginger root

4 cups Quick Vegetable Stock (page 266) or store-bought vegetable broth

2 tablespoons shiro (white) miso, or more to taste

Sea salt, to taste (optional)

2 scallions, white and light green parts only, thinly sliced

1. Heat the oils in a 2-quart saucepan over medium heat. Add the onion, carrot, and ginger and cook, stirring frequently, until the onion is translucent. Add the broth and bring to a boil, then reduce the heat to low. Cover and simmer until the carrot is barely tender, about 6 to 8 minutes. Remove from the heat and discard the ginger.

2. Put about ½ tablespoon of miso in each bowl, then ladle in about ½ cup of the broth. Stir to dissolve the miso. Add another ½ cup of the broth to each bowl. Taste and adjust the seasoning, adding more miso or a bit of salt if needed. Garnish with scallions and serve.

CARROT and PARSNIP SOUP

SERVES 6, **VEG, V*, GF**

Carrots and parsnips are a natural pairing, both root vegetables with their own sweetness and distinctive tastes. Most people will think of this as a warming soup to enjoy in fall or winter, but it is also quite good cold when the weather is hot.

2 tablespoons grapeseed oil

6 carrots (about 1 pound), peeled, halved lengthwise, and cut into thin half-moons

4 parsnips (about 1 pound), peeled, halved lengthwise, and cut into thin half-moons

Sea salt, to taste

Pinch of crushed red pepper flakes, or more to taste

2 tablespoons extra-virgin olive oil

2 shallots, finely chopped

4 garlic cloves, pressed and allowed to sit for 10 minutes

1 tablespoon finely chopped fresh thyme leaves or 1 teaspoon dried thyme

6 cups Quick Vegetable Stock (page 266) or store-bought vegetable broth

1 tablespoon balsamic vinegar

¼ cup chopped fresh chives

1 cup plain Greek yogurt (optional)

1. Heat the grapeseed oil in a soup pot over medium-high heat and sauté the carrots and parsnips. Season them with salt and red pepper flakes and cook, stirring often, for 10 minutes or until lightly browned.

2. Reduce the heat to low and pour in the olive oil. Stir in the shallots, garlic, and thyme and sauté until the shallots and garlic just begin to brown, about 4 to 5 minutes.

3. Turn the heat to high and pour in the stock. Bring the soup to a simmer, reduce the heat to medium, and cook for 5 to 6 minutes or until the carrots are tender. Add the vinegar and blend the soup directly in the pot with an immersion blender. Taste and adjust the seasoning, adding more salt, red pepper flakes, or vinegar, if necessary.

4. Garnish each bowl with the chives and a dollop of plain Greek yogurt.

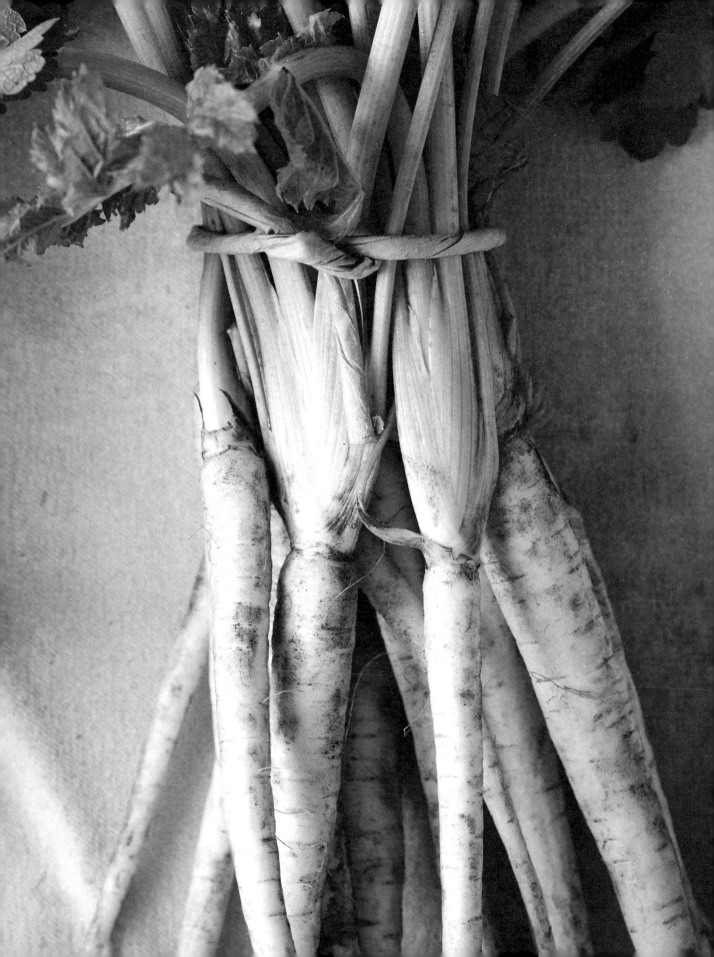

ROASTED RED PEPPER SOUP

SERVES 6, **VEG**, **V***, **GF**

Roasted red peppers give a bright color and velvety texture to this soup, which is highly flavored with garlic, cumin, lime, and cilantro. You could blacken red bell peppers over a gas flame or on a grill, then seal them in a paper bag to loosen the skins and peel and seed them, but that takes time and patience. Or you can buy jarred roasted, peeled, and seeded red peppers, which work just fine in this soup. The sautéed corn makes a lovely finishing touch.

3 tablespoons extra-virgin olive oil, plus more for finishing

1 onion, chopped

2 garlic cloves, pressed and allowed to sit for 10 minutes

½ teaspoon ground cumin

⅛ teaspoon crushed red pepper flakes

Sea salt, to taste

2 (12-ounce) jars roasted red peppers, drained and roughly chopped

2 teaspoons grade B maple syrup

4 to 5 cups Quick Vegetable Stock (page 266) or store-bought vegetable broth

1½ cups frozen supersweet corn

½ teaspoon grated lime zest

2 teaspoons lime juice

¼ cup fresh cilantro leaves, finely chopped

¼ cup crumbled queso fresco or feta cheese (optional)

Lime wedges

1. In a soup pot heat 2 tablespoons of the oil over medium-high heat and sauté the onion until translucent. Add the garlic, cumin, red pepper flakes, and a pinch of salt and sauté for 3 minutes more. Stir in the roasted peppers, maple syrup, and broth and increase the heat to high. When the soup begins to bubble, cover the pot, reduce the heat to low, and let it simmer for 10 to 15 minutes.

2. Meanwhile, in a small skillet, heat the remaining 1 tablespoon oil over medium-high heat. Add the frozen corn, season it with salt, and cook, stirring occasionally, for 5 minutes. Turn off the heat and stir in the lime zest, lime juice, and two-thirds of the cilantro; transfer to a bowl and allow to cool.

3. Blend the soup directly in the pot with an immersion blender until completely smooth. Taste and adjust seasoning, if necessary, with more salt or lime juice.

4. To serve, garnish each bowl with corn, cheese, a drizzle of good quality extra-virgin olive oil, and a lime wedge on the side.

MUSHROOM BARLEY SOUP

SERVES 8, **V**

Mushroom Barley Soup is a traditional winter soup often associated with Eastern Europe that can be made both with meat (usually beef) and without. This vegan version gets its deep flavor from porcini and shiitake mushrooms, wine, and herbs. The chewy barley makes it filling. It's too bad that this ancient grain, the original source of malt for beer and flour for bread in Tibet, is largely neglected in North America. It is quite tasty and, unlike most grains, has a lot of soluble fiber, which lowers its glycemic index. (Barley does contain gluten.) Although the grain takes time to cook, the preparation of this soup is quick.

½ ounce dried porcini mushrooms

½ ounce dried shiitake mushrooms

3 tablespoons extra-virgin olive oil

1 yellow onion, diced

1 teaspoon plus a pinch of sea salt

¾ pound mushrooms, sliced

1 carrot, peeled and diced

1 celery stalk, sliced

2 garlic cloves, pressed and allowed to sit for 10 minutes

1 teaspoon dried thyme or
1 tablespoon minced fresh thyme

½ cup dry vermouth

4 cups Quick Vegetable Stock (page 266) or store-bought vegetable broth

½ cup pearl barley

½ teaspoon freshly ground black pepper

3 tablespoons chopped fresh flat-leaf parsley leaves

1. In a 2-quart saucepan, bring 4 cups of water to a boil, then add the dried mushrooms. Turn off the heat, cover, and let soak for 20 minutes. Strain the mushrooms through a fine-mesh sieve over a bowl to remove the sediment, reserving the liquid. Remove and discard the stems. Finely chop the mushroom caps and set aside.

2. In a Dutch oven or soup pot, heat the olive oil over medium-high heat. Add the onions and a pinch of salt. Stir and cook for about 4 minutes. Add the fresh mushrooms, carrots, celery, and ½ teaspoon of the salt. Stir and cook until vegetables begin to get tender, 5 to 6 minutes. Add the garlic and thyme and stir to combine.

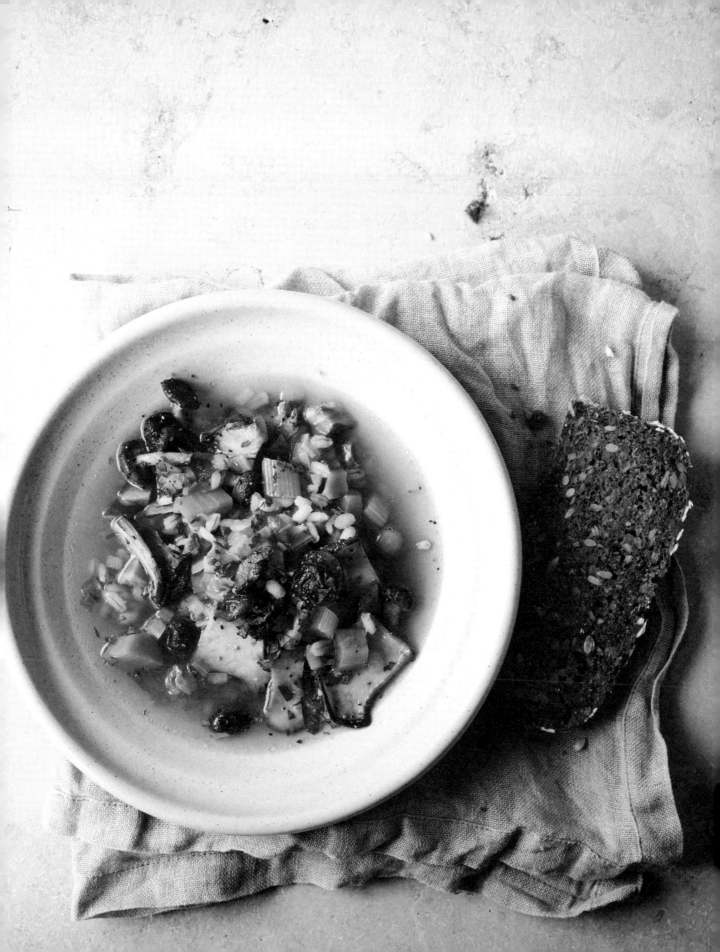

3. Add the vermouth to deglaze the pot. Stir until the liquid has reduced by half, about 3 minutes, then add the soaked dried mushrooms, mushroom water, stock, barley, remaining ½ teaspoon salt, and pepper. Bring to a simmer, reduce the heat, and cook for 40 to 45 minutes or until the barley is tender.

4. To serve, garnish each bowl with parsley.

TORTILLA SOUP with SHRIMP

SERVES 4 TO 6

This quick version of the popular Mexican soup can be paired with a salad to make a simple meal. Instead of frying the tortillas, you bake them after brushing them with olive oil and seasoning them. They soften in the spicy broth, adding a chewy textural contrast to the firmer shrimp and soft avocado. Fresh lime juice adds a bright finish.

3 corn tortillas, cut into strips

4 tablespoons extra-virgin olive oil

½ teaspoon ground cumin

½ teaspoon mild red chili powder

½ teaspoon sea salt

4 garlic cloves, pressed and allowed to sit for 10 minutes

1 pound raw shrimp, peeled and deveined, shells reserved

3 flat-leaf parsley sprigs

Freshly ground black pepper, to taste

5 cups Quick Vegetable Stock (page 266) or store-bought vegetable broth

1 onion, chopped

1 cup diced fresh tomatoes, drained, or 1 cup canned tomatoes, seeded and drained

1 jalapeño pepper, seeded and halved lengthwise

1 tablespoon chopped fresh oregano or 1½ teaspoons dried oregano

⅓ cup lime juice

¼ cup chopped fresh cilantro leaves, plus more for garnish

1 avocado

Lime wedges

¼ cup finely chopped red onion (optional)

1. Preheat the oven to 375°F and line a rimmed baking sheet with parchment paper.

2. Brush the tortillas with 1 tablespoon of the oil and sprinkle them with cumin, chili powder, and ¼ teaspoon of salt. Place the tortillas on the baking sheet and bake for 8 minutes or until crisp, flipping them once after 4 minutes.

3. Heat 2 tablespoons of the oil in a soup pot over medium heat and sauté ¼ of the garlic with the shrimp shells and parsley. Season with the remaining ¼ teaspoon salt and black pepper and cook for 2 to 3 minutes. Pour in the broth and turn the heat to high. Once the broth comes to a boil, reduce the heat and simmer for about 5 minutes. Strain the broth through a fine-mesh

strainer into a heatproof bowl and firmly press on the shells to squeeze out their flavor. Discard the shells and set broth aside.

4. Heat the remaining 1 tablespoon oil in the pot over medium heat and sauté the onion for 4 to 5 minutes until it's soft. Add the tomatoes, jalapeño, remaining garlic, and oregano and cook for 3 to 4 minutes. Add the shrimp and let cook until opaque and just barely cooked through, about 1 minute. Increase the heat to high and pour in the shrimp broth. Stir in the lime juice and ¼ cup cilantro. As soon as the broth has warmed through, taste and adjust the seasoning with more salt, pepper, or lime, if necessary.

5. Divide the tortilla strips evenly among 4 to 6 bowls and ladle the soup over them. Garnish with a few pieces of avocado in the center of each bowl and serve with lime wedges, additional cilantro, and red onion, if desired, on the side.

TUSCAN BEAN SOUP
with FARRO and SWISS CHARD

SERVES 6, **VEG**

This version of a classic main-dish soup from Tuscany makes use of canned white beans to save time. You can use Tuscan kale in place of chard if you wish. I like to serve this with extra grated Parmesan and red pepper flakes on the side as well as a cruet of very flavorful olive oil for guests to drizzle over the soup.

3 tablespoons extra-virgin olive oil

1 onion, diced

½ teaspoon plus a pinch of sea salt

4 cloves garlic, pressed and allowed to sit for 10 minutes

Generous pinch of crushed red pepper flakes

3 tablespoons tomato paste

½ bunch Swiss chard, stems removed and chopped into bite-size pieces, leaves torn into bite-size pieces

1 tablespoon minced fresh thyme or 1 teaspoon dried thyme

1 teaspoon minced fresh rosemary or ¼ teaspoon dried rosemary

1 Turkish bay leaf or ⅓ of a California bay leaf

1 (14.5-ounce) can diced tomatoes, drained and juices reserved

8 cups Quick Vegetable Stock (page 266) or store-bought vegetable broth

¾ cup cooked farro (page 196)

1 (15-ounce) can cannellini or great northern beans, rinsed and drained

2 tablespoons chopped fresh flat-leaf parsley leaves

1 tablespoon chopped fresh oregano

1 teaspoon lemon juice

Freshly ground black pepper

Shaved Parmesan cheese

1. Heat the olive oil in a soup pot over medium heat. Add the onion and a pinch of salt and sauté until the onions are golden, about 4 minutes. Add the garlic and red pepper flakes and sauté for another 30 seconds. Push the onions and garlic to the side and sauté the tomato paste for about 1 minute. Add the chard stems, thyme, rosemary, and bay leaf, stirring to combine.

2. Pour in the reserved tomato juice to deglaze the pot and cook until the liquid is reduced by half, about 2 minutes. Add the diced tomatoes, stock, and remaining ½ teaspoon salt. Increase the heat to high and bring to a boil.

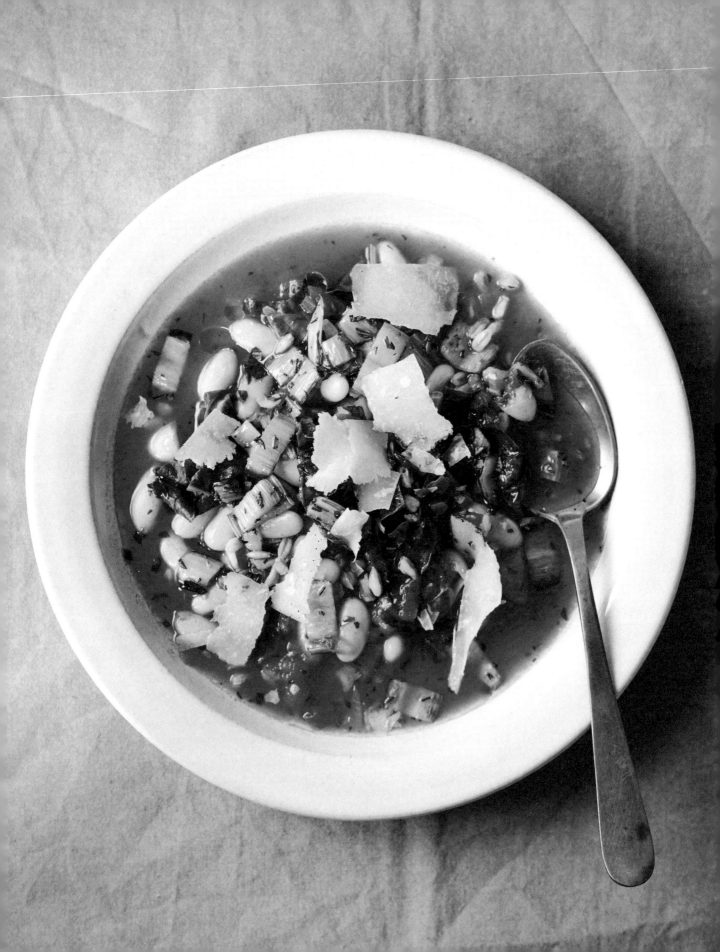

3. Reduce the heat to medium-low and add the farro and beans. Cook for another 3 minutes, until the beans and farro are heated through.

4. Stir in the chard leaves, parsley, oregano, and lemon juice. Adjust the seasoning with black pepper and another pinch or two of salt, if needed, and garnish each bowl with a generous shaving of Parmesan cheese.

VEGETABLE MINESTRONE with QUINOA

SERVES 4 TO 6, **VEG, V*, GF**

Minestrone is a vegetable soup of ancient Italian origin made from whatever vegetables are in season, sometimes with meat or beans and often including pasta or rice. Tomatoes, being native to the New World, are a late addition to the mix. Minestrone is a thick and filling soup that can be a main course. This version gets a big flavor boost from the garlic oil and basil added just before serving.

¼ cup extra-virgin olive oil

12 garlic cloves, pressed and allowed to sit for 10 minutes

1 leek, trimmed, thinly sliced

2 carrots, peeled and roughly chopped

2 celery stalks, roughly chopped

Sea salt and freshly ground black pepper, to taste

¼ teaspoon crushed red pepper flakes

2 zucchini, cut into ¼-inch half-moons

1 (14.5-ounce) can chopped tomatoes

4 to 5 cups Quick Vegetable Stock (page 266) or store-bought vegetable broth

1 bunch Swiss chard, stemmed and roughly chopped

1 cup quinoa, rinsed

½ cup finely sliced fresh basil leaves

Freshly grated Parmesan cheese

1. Heat 2 tablespoons of the oil in large soup pot over medium heat and sauté half the garlic and the leek until softened, about 3 to 5 minutes. Add the carrots and celery and season with a large pinch of salt, some black pepper, and the red pepper flakes.

2. Cook the vegetables, stirring occasionally, until they soften slightly. Transfer the cooked vegetables to a bowl and set aside. Raise the heat slightly and add the zucchini. Season the zucchini with salt, cook on each side until browned, and add to the bowl of mixed vegetables.

3. Turn the heat to high and add the tomatoes; cook for 2 to 3 minutes, then pour in the broth and bring up to a slow boil. Add the sautéed vegetables back to the pot along with the Swiss chard and the quinoa. Cook for 10 to 15 minutes or until the quinoa is tender.

4. Heat the remaining 2 tablespoons olive oil in a small sauté pan and quickly sauté the remaining garlic with a pinch of salt and red pepper flakes until aromatic. Add the garlic oil and basil to the minestrone. Taste and adjust seasoning with salt, if necessary. Garnish each bowl with freshly grated Parmesan cheese.

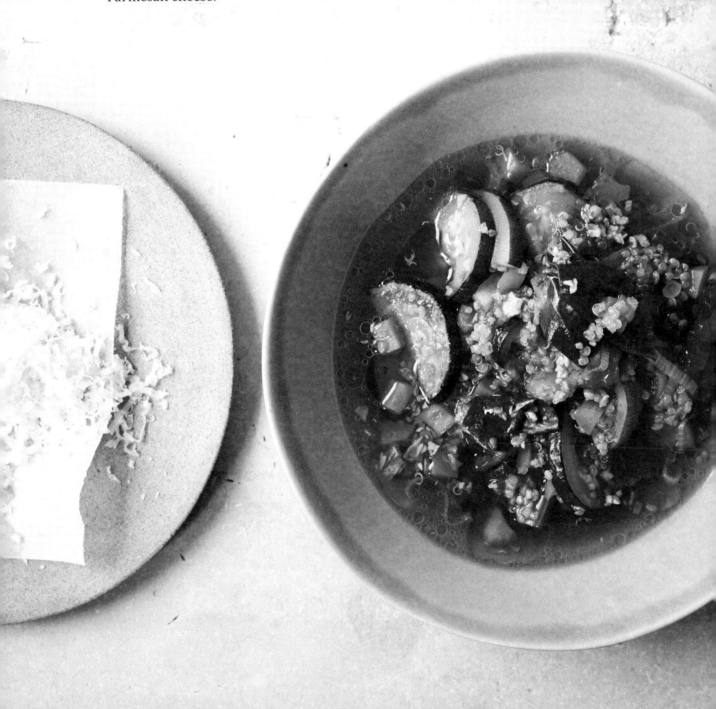

WINTER ROOT SOUP

SERVES 8, **VEG, V*, GF**

This deeply flavored, nourishing soup is one you might expect to find on the table of a European farmhouse on a cold winter night. It is totally satisfying without being overly rich and is a snap to cook once the root vegetables are peeled and cut. To my taste, the flavor combination of olive oil, garlic, dry vermouth, and freshly grated Parmesan cheese is irresistible. Serve this with a green salad for a simple, rustic meal.

2 tablespoons extra-virgin olive oil

1 large onion, diced

2 Yukon gold potatoes, peeled and cut into bite-size pieces

2 parsnips, peeled and cut into bite-size pieces

2 large carrots, peeled and cut into bite-size pieces

1 rutabaga, peeled and cut into bite-size pieces

1 turnip, peeled and cut into bite-size pieces

2 garlic cloves, pressed and allowed to sit for 10 minutes

½ teaspoon dried thyme

½ teaspoon dried marjoram

½ teaspoon dried basil

Sea salt and freshly ground black pepper, to taste

1 cup dry (white) vermouth

4 to 5 cups Quick Vegetable Broth (page 266) or store-bought vegetable broth

1 Turkish bay leaf or ⅓ of a California bay leaf

1 bunch fresh flat-leaf parsley, leaves picked and chopped

1 cup freshly grated Parmesan cheese

1. Heat the oil in soup pot over medium heat, add the onion, and sauté for 4 to 5 minutes or until translucent.

2. Increase the heat slightly and add the root vegetables, stirring occasionally, until they are browned on the edges, about 5 to 6 minutes. Add the garlic, thyme, marjoram, and basil and continue to cook for one more minute.

3. Season with a generous pinch of both salt and black pepper, then pour in the vermouth. Gently scrape the bottom of the pan with a wooden spoon to lift any browned bits of vegetables. Pour in the stock, add the bay leaf, and

bring the soup to a boil, then reduce the heat so the soup is simmering. Cook for 8 to 10 minutes or until the vegetables are just tender.

4. Remove from heat. Taste and adjust with more salt or pepper, if necessary, and remove the bay leaf. Garnish each bowl with the chopped parsley and grated Parmesan cheese.

YAM and PEANUT SOUP

SERVES 8, **V, GF**

There are many ways of making this hearty soup, inspired by African cuisine (although yams, tomatoes, and both sweet and hot peppers are all native to the New World). I first tasted a version at a creative vegetarian restaurant in Victoria, British Columbia, the much-loved Rebar Modern Food. (I highly recommend the *Rebar: Modern Food Cookbook*.) Many people will find the combinations of flavors in this soup novel and appealing. This is a good first course for fall and winter.

1 tablespoon grapeseed oil

½ large yellow onion, diced

½ teaspoon sea salt, or more to taste

2 garlic cloves, pressed and allowed to sit for 10 minutes

3 tablespoons peeled, finely grated fresh ginger

1½ teaspoons ground cumin

1½ teaspoons ground coriander

½ teaspoon sweet paprika

¼ teaspoon cayenne pepper

2 yams, peeled and cut into ½-inch cubes

1 small red bell pepper, seeded and diced

4 cups Quick Vegetable Stock (page 266) or store-bought vegetable broth

½ cup freshly squeezed orange juice

1 large ripe tomato, chopped, or ⅓ cup canned diced plum tomatoes

2½ tablespoons natural smooth peanut butter

¼ cup dry-roasted peanuts, chopped

½ cup fresh cilantro leaves, chopped (optional)

2 limes, quartered

Hot sauce, to taste

1. Heat the oil in a large soup pot over medium-high heat. Add the onions and a pinch of salt and sauté until translucent, about 6 minutes. Add the garlic, ginger, and spices, and sauté for 2 minutes more.

2. Reduce the heat to medium, add the yams and red pepper, and sauté until they start to just stick to the bottom of the pot, about 4 to 5 minutes.

3. Add 3 cups of the stock, the orange juice, tomato, and peanut butter and stir to combine. Bring the soup to a boil and then reduce the heat so it is simmering. Cover and cook until the yams are tender, about 15 minutes.

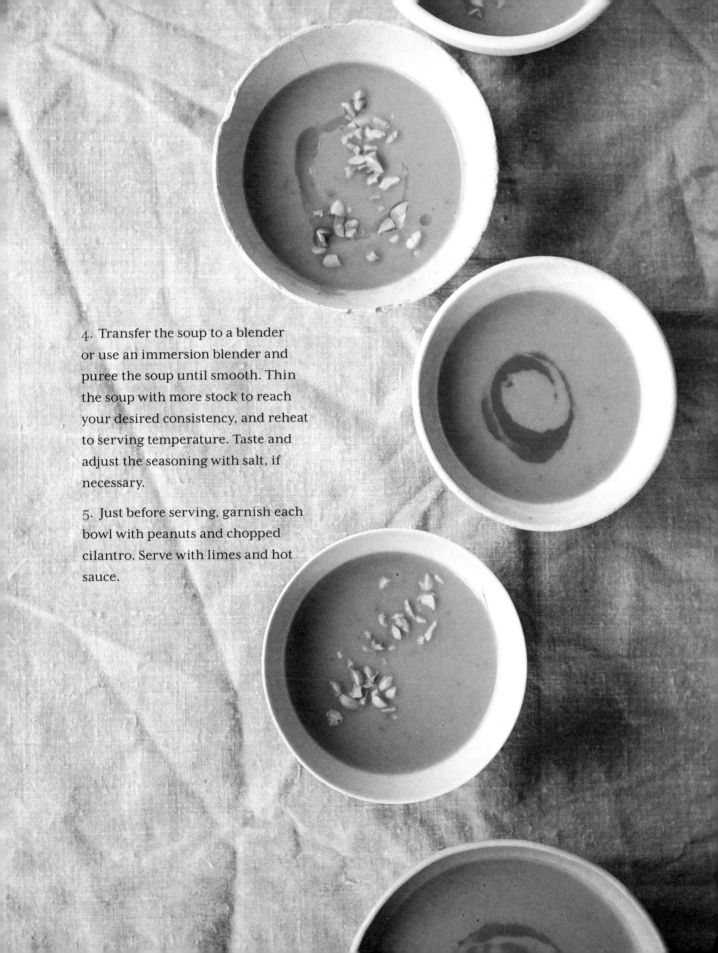

4. Transfer the soup to a blender or use an immersion blender and puree the soup until smooth. Thin the soup with more stock to reach your desired consistency, and reheat to serving temperature. Taste and adjust the seasoning with salt, if necessary.

5. Just before serving, garnish each bowl with peanuts and chopped cilantro. Serve with limes and hot sauce.

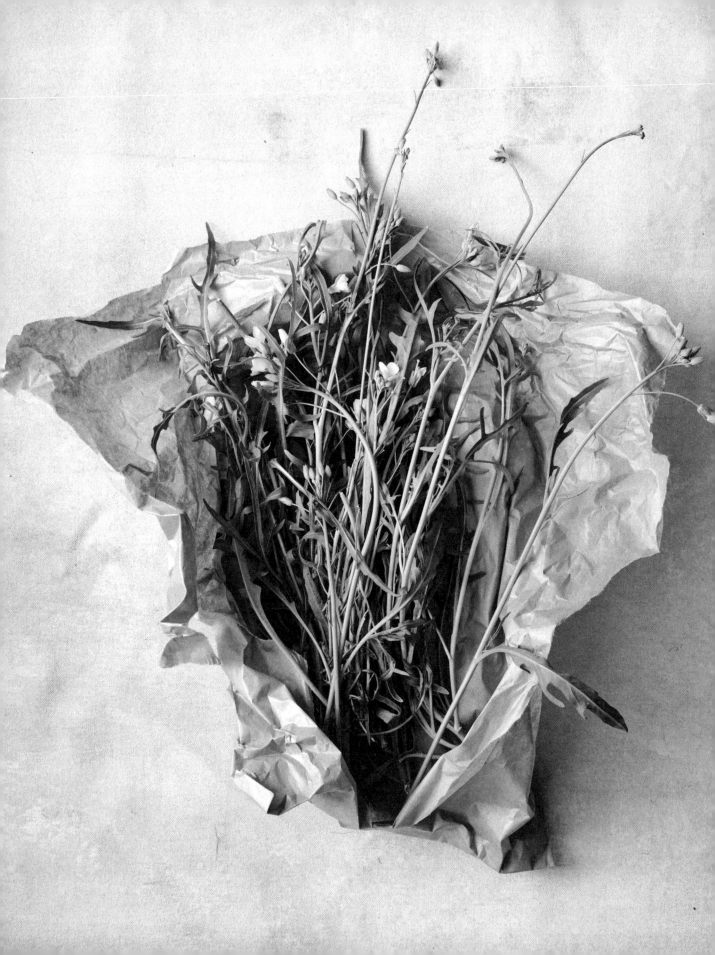

Salads

So many different dishes are called salad that it's hard to know what the term means. Many salads consist of raw leafy vegetables served cold or at room temperature with a dressing, but others have cooked vegetables, grains, nuts, fruit, cheese, seafood, or meats. They are usually served before, with, or after main courses of meals but can be substantial enough to stand on their own. Japanese and some Middle Easterners eat salad for breakfast. (So do I.) If there is one unifying quality of salads, it seems to be temperature: almost all of them are cold or cool. *Warm salad* is an oxymoron (even though you may encounter one). Because freshness is a large part of their appeal, salads should be put on the table soon after you make them; however, many of the ingredients in the recipes that follow can be prepped in advance for easy assembly. The range of salad possibilities here will, I hope, inspire you to try out variations and creations of your own.

Recipes marked **veg** are vegetarian, those marked **v** are vegan, and those marked **gf** are gluten-free. The symbols **veg***, **v***, and **gf*** indicate recipes that can be modified to be vegetarian, vegan, or gluten-free by substituting or omitting specific ingredients.

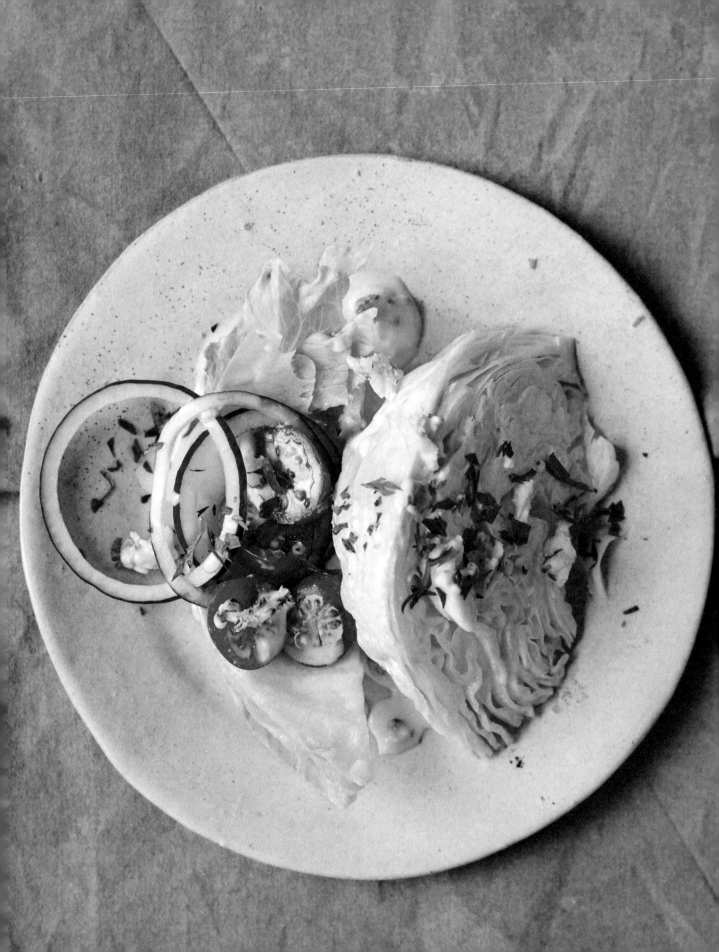

ICEBERG WEDGE, RED ONION, and TOMATO
with BLUE CHEESE DRESSING

SERVES 4, **VEG, GF**

For years, it has not been politically correct to like iceberg lettuce, a variety supposed to be lacking in nutrients, the vegetable equivalent of white bread. I've always loved iceberg for its distinctive crunch, unmatched by any other lettuce. I grow it in my garden and assure you that fresh, garden-grown iceberg is a real treat, full of flavor as well as crunch. Now I grow a new type, red iceberg, that I hope will soon appear in farmers' markets and, eventually, in supermarkets. It's beautiful and rich in beneficial phytonutrients. One of my favorite ways to enjoy it is to pour a great blue cheese dressing over a chilled, crisp wedge.

DRESSING Makes 1 cup

½ cup crumbled blue cheese

1 (7-ounce) container or ¾ cup plain Greek yogurt

2 tablespoons mayonnaise

1½ teaspoons Worcestershire sauce

1 tablespoon milk

½ teaspoon apple cider vinegar

¼ teaspoon sea salt

¼ teaspoon freshly ground black pepper

¼ teaspoon grade B maple syrup

SALAD

1 large head iceberg lettuce, trimmed and quartered

¼ cup thinly sliced red onion

12 cherry tomatoes, halved

2 tablespoons coarsely chopped fresh flat-leaf parsley leaves

1. Place ¼ cup of the blue cheese and all of the other dressing ingredients into a blender, and blend on medium speed until smooth.

2. Transfer the dressing to a bowl and whisk in the remaining blue cheese; refrigerate until ready to use.

3. Dress each lettuce wedge with a few tablespoons of blue cheese dressing and top each portion with onion, tomatoes, and chopped parsley. Store extra dressing in an airtight container in the refrigerator for up to 1 week.

BASIC GREEN SALAD

SERVES 4, **V, GF**

Too often, when I order salad out, the dressing is sweet and there's too much of it. Instead of just greens, I get concoctions of fruits, nuts, goat cheese, and more. There is a time and place for these, but sometimes a simple salad is just the thing. The French know how to make a basic green salad that is a snap to prepare. Dry leaves are critical here—there's nothing worse than a soggy salad. Don't overdress it. Feel free to get rid of the salad tongs and use your hands to toss the greens; you get more air into your mix that way, allowing for better incorporation of the vinaigrette. Salad greens can be washed and spun in advance, then wrapped in tea towels, placed in vegetable storage bags, and kept in the refrigerator for several days.

1 head romaine lettuce, torn into pieces

1 head butter lettuce, large leaves torn

2 teaspoons chopped fresh flat-leaf parsley leaves

Pinch of sea salt

Freshly ground black pepper

½ cup **Basic French Vinaigrette** (page 267)

1. Place the lettuce leaves and the parsley in a large salad bowl and season with a pinch of sea salt and a few grinds of pepper.

2. Drizzle the dressing along the walls of your bowl, then lightly toss the greens (with your hands, if you like) until the dressing is evenly distributed. Serve the salad from a bowl or transfer to 4 individual plates.

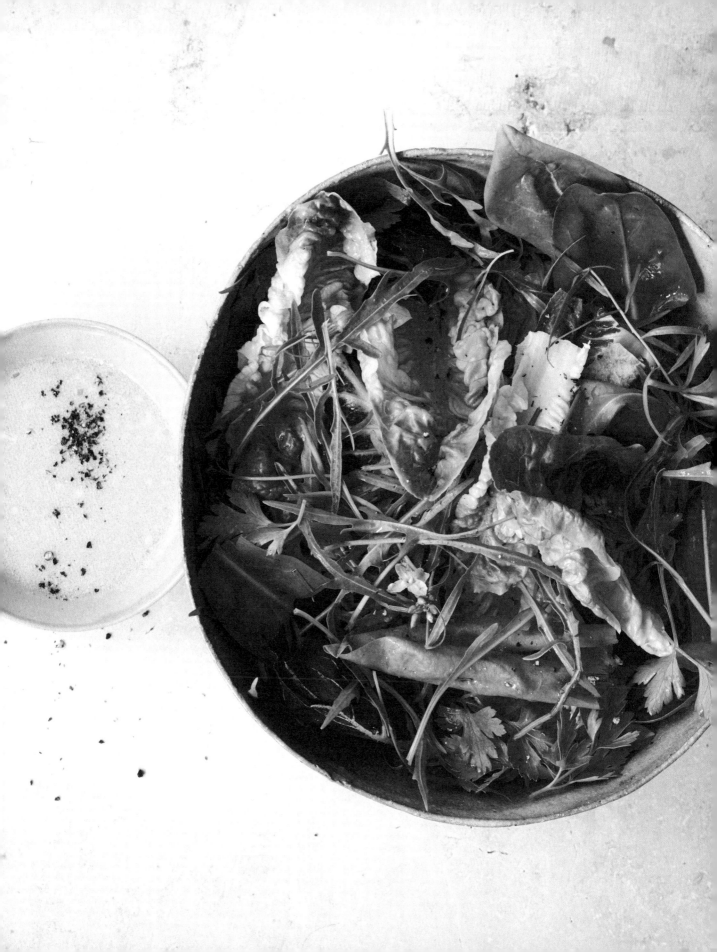

WATERMELON CUCUMBER SALAD
with TOASTED PISTACHIOS and FETA

SERVES 4, **V***, **GF**

One word for this: *refreshing.* Or two words: *very refreshing.* A super-hydrating treat for the summer months, and beautiful too. The antioxidant and anti-inflammatory properties of watermelon increase as the fruit ripens. Look for heavy, firm, and symmetrical melons that have dark green skins and yellow underbellies and that sound hollow when you give them a knock.

DRESSING

1 teaspoon grated lime zest

2 tablespoons lime juice

½ teaspoon sea salt

⅛ teaspoon freshly ground black pepper

1 teaspoon grade B maple syrup

¼ cup extra-virgin olive oil

SALAD

½ small watermelon, peeled, seeded, and cut into ¾-inch cubes (about 2 cups)

1 small English cucumber, peeled, seeded, and cut into ½-inch dice

2 tablespoons torn fresh spearmint

2 tablespoons chopped toasted pistachios

1 tablespoon crumbled feta cheese (optional)

1. Place the lime zest, lime juice, salt, pepper, and maple syrup together in a large bowl and whisk to combine. Drizzle in the olive oil, whisking until fully combined.

2. Add the watermelon, cucumber, and spearmint to the dressing and toss until well coated. Just before serving, garnish each portion with pistachios and feta cheese.

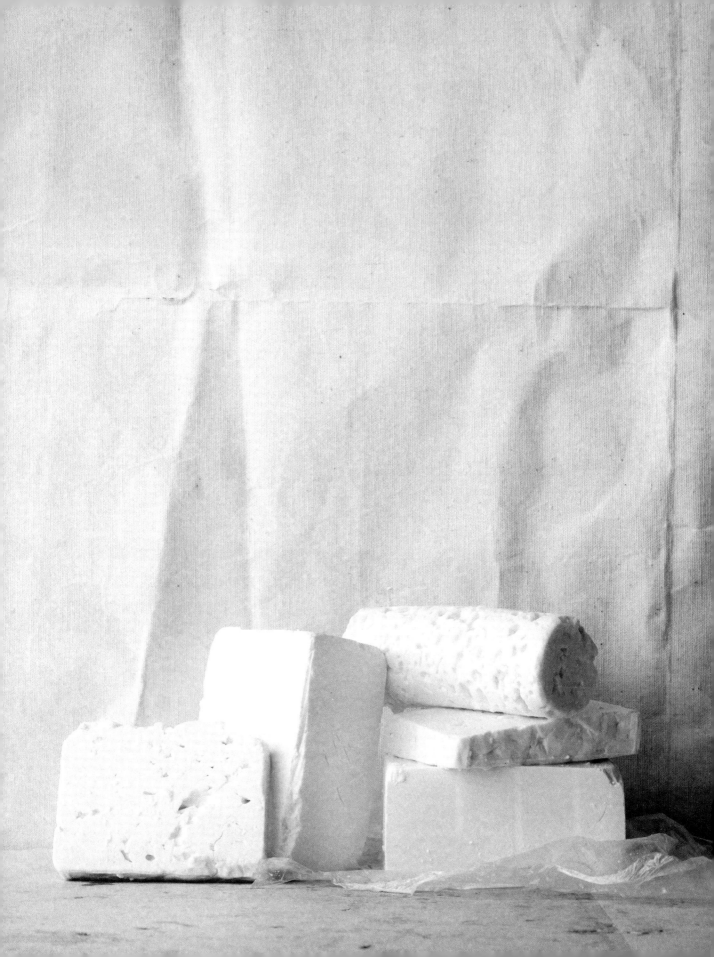

GREEK-STYLE KALE SALAD

SERVES 4, **VEG, GF**

A novel but logical twist on a raw kale salad. Marinating the leaves in the dressing softens and debitters them while the dressing changes their color from bluish green to green. If you are in a hurry, you can hasten the process by massaging the dressing into the kale with your fingers. (It's fun to do this even if you're not in a hurry.) It's remarkable how well this most nutritious vegetable goes with the other ingredients and flavors of a typical Greek salad.

1 small red onion, halved and thinly sliced

Dash of lemon juice or vinegar

⅓ cup Basic Lemon Vinaigrette (page 267), plus more if needed

1 bunch black kale (also called Tuscan or lacinato kale or cavolo nero), ribs removed and leaves torn into bite-size pieces

1 pint cherry tomatoes, halved

1 cucumber, halved, quartered lengthwise, seeded, and cut into ½-inch pieces

½ cup halved, pitted Kalamata olives

¼ cup crumbled feta cheese

1. Place the sliced onions in a small bowl and cover them with water and a spritz of lemon juice or vinegar. Allow them to sit for 10 minutes, then drain. (This renders them less sharp.)

2. Add the dressing to a large bowl. Add the kale and toss well to coat. Allow the dressed kale to sit at room temperature for 10 to 30 minutes. Add the onions, cherry tomatoes, cucumber, and olives and toss again, adding more dressing if you like. Transfer the salad to a serving platter and top with feta cheese.

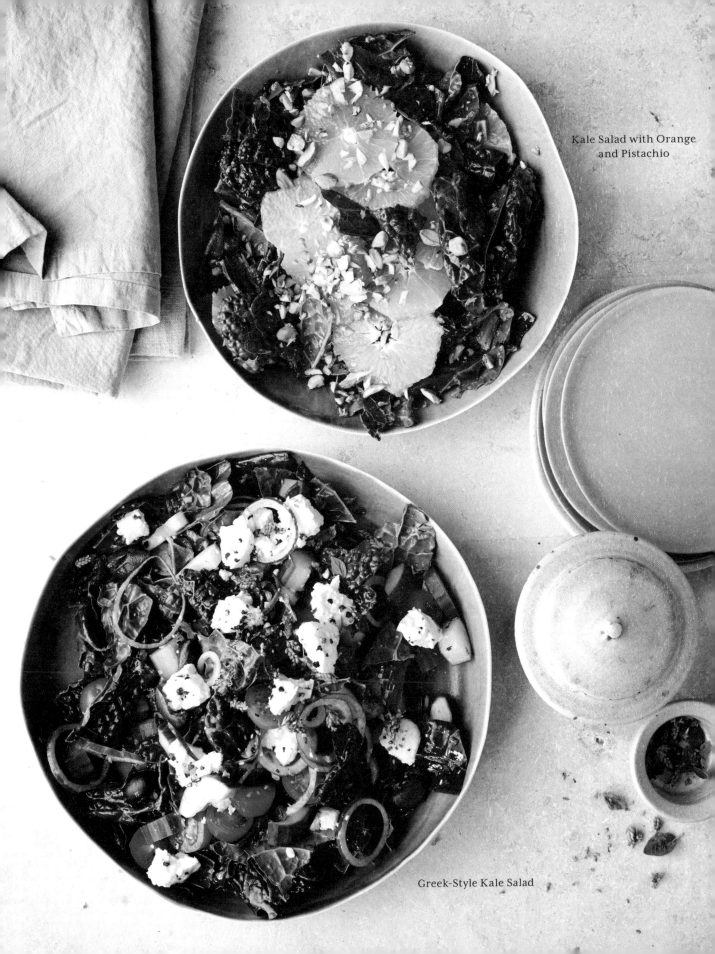

Kale Salad with Orange
and Pistachio

Greek-Style Kale Salad

KALE SALAD with ORANGE and PISTACHIO

SERVES 4, **V, GF**

This is unlike any kale salad you have ever had. The natural sweetness of dates (also full of fiber) contrasts with the sour taste of citrus and slight bitterness of kale, all balanced and harmonized by the warming spices. As with any kale salad, it is important to allow the leaves to soften in texture and flavor through contact with lemon juice and salt. If you can't wait 30 minutes for this process, you can speed it up by massaging the dressing into the kale before you add the dates.

DRESSING

¼ cup extra-virgin olive oil

3 tablespoons lemon juice

1 teaspoon orange zest

1 tablespoon orange juice

½ teaspoon sea salt

½ teaspoon ground cumin

⅛ teaspoon ground cinnamon

⅛ teaspoon cayenne pepper

SALAD

1 bunch black kale (also called Tuscan or lacinato kale or cavolo nero), ribs removed and leaves torn into bite-size pieces

½ cup pitted and coarsely chopped dates

2 blood or Valencia oranges, peeled and cut crosswise into circles

¼ cup raw pistachios, toasted (page 274)

1. In a large bowl, whisk together the dressing ingredients until well combined.

2. Add the kale and dates and toss well to coat. Let the salad sit at room temperature for 10 to 30 minutes.

3. Transfer the salad to a serving platter, add the oranges, and top with the toasted pistachios.

MEDITERRANEAN SARDINES
over FENNEL and ARUGULA

SERVES 4, **GF**

Sardines are one of the best sources of the omega-3 fatty acids we need. They are also inexpensive, readily available, and sustainable; in fact, there is a great abundance of sardines in the world today, one of the few choice wild-fish populations not in decline. If you don't like sardines, I'm not going to tell you that this recipe will change your mind, but I think the mustardy vinaigrette and herbs nicely offset their fishiness.

DRESSING

2 tablespoons lemon juice

1 teaspoon Dijon mustard

1 tablespoon minced shallot

½ teaspoon sea salt

⅛ teaspoon freshly ground black pepper

¼ cup extra-virgin olive oil

½ cup chopped tomatoes

2 teaspoons rinsed and drained chopped capers

2 teaspoons finely chopped fresh oregano or ¾ teaspoon dried oregano

SALAD

3 bunches (about 6 cups) arugula

¼ cup fresh flat-leaf parsley leaves

2 fennel bulbs, thinly sliced (about 2 cups)

2 to 3 (5-ounce) cans boneless, skinless sardines packed in water

1 avocado, sliced

1. Put the lemon juice, Dijon mustard, shallot, salt, and pepper in a small bowl and whisk to combine. Slowly pour in the olive oil, whisking all the while, and continue whisking until smooth, or blend all the ingredients in a jar with the solid disk of an immersion blender. Add the tomatoes, capers, and oregano and stir to combine.

2. Combine the arugula, parsley, and fennel in a large bowl and toss with ½ cup of the dressing. Divide the greens evenly among 4 plates and top each portion with some sardines.

3. Spoon 1 tablespoon of the remaining dressing over the top of the sardines. Divide the avocado slices among the plates and serve. (Store extra dressing in a jar in the refrigerator for up to 3 days.)

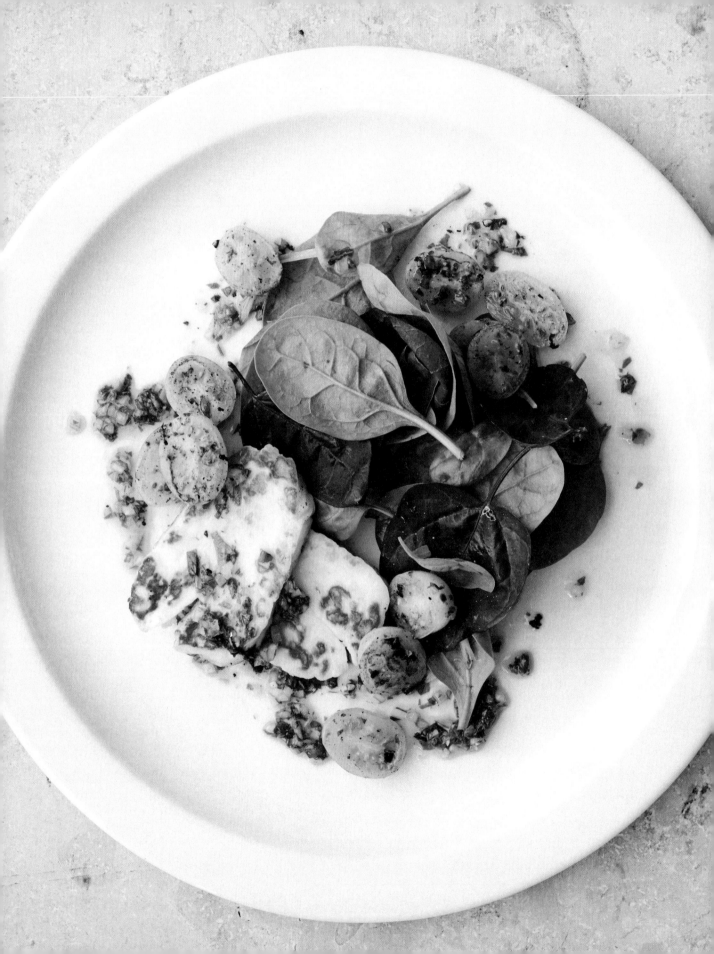

GRILLED HALLOUMI and TOMATO SALAD

SERVES 4, **VEG, GF**

Halloumi is a semi-hard cheese, native to the island of Cyprus, made from goat's milk, sheep's milk, cow's milk, or some combination. I prefer the pure sheep's milk version. Halloumi comes packed in brine and is best grilled or lightly browned without oil in a nonstick skillet. Eaten within minutes of cooking, it is warm and a bit chewy with a delicious flavor. You can put strips or chunks of grilled halloumi on any salad. Try it for breakfast. I also like it rolled into a wrap with lettuce, tomato, and onion and a bit of olive oil and red wine vinegar dressing.

DRESSING

3 garlic cloves, pressed and allowed to sit for 10 minutes

2 small shallots, roughly chopped

2 tablespoons lemon juice

1 tablespoon white wine vinegar

½ teaspoon sea salt

¼ cup extra-virgin olive oil

¼ cup chopped fresh spearmint

¾ cup chopped fresh basil

SALAD

2 pints cherry or grape tomatoes

16 ounces halloumi, sliced into ½-inch-thick slabs

½ pound or ½ bag (about 3 cups) prepacked spinach

3 tablespoons sliced spearmint

3 tablespoons sliced fresh basil

1. Preheat the oven to 475°F and line a rimmed baking sheet with parchment paper.

2. Blend the dressing ingredients in a blender or with the solid disk of an immersion blender until smooth, and set aside.

3. Put the tomatoes in a bowl, toss with 2 tablespoons of the dressing, and place on the baking sheet. Roast the tomatoes for 10 minutes or until they're bursting and lightly charred.

4. Meanwhile, heat a nonstick pan over medium heat. When the pan is hot, add the slices of cheese. Cook for 1 to 2 minutes, then turn them and continue cooking for another minute on the other side until both sides are golden brown.

5. Place the spinach on a large serving platter, and when the cheese and tomatoes are done, arrange them attractively on top. Drizzle over the remaining dressing and garnish with the spearmint and basil. Serve while the cheese is still melted and hot.

LENTIL TABBOULEH

SERVES 6, **V, GF**

Lentils rarely get their due in our part of the world. These humble legumes are prized in other cultures—they are inexpensive, protein-rich, and great blood-sugar stabilizers. Here, I've used lentils instead of bulgur wheat or another grain to make a satisfying tabbouleh. This easy side can go with anything.

LENTILS

1 cup dried lentils, preferably Le Puy green lentils, rinsed well

2 garlic cloves, pressed and allowed to sit for 10 minutes

1 Turkish bay leaf or ⅓ of a California bay leaf

¼ teaspoon sea salt

½ cup Basic Lemon Vinaigrette (page 267)

SALAD

1 small cucumber, peeled, seeded, and diced small

12 cherry tomatoes, halved

¼ cup chopped fresh spearmint

½ cup chopped fresh flat-leaf parsley leaves

¼ teaspoon sea salt

Freshly ground black pepper

Dash of lemon juice

1. Combine the lentils, garlic, and bay leaf in a saucepan and cover with 2 cups of water. Bring to a boil, then cover, lower the heat, and simmer for 15 minutes. Stir the salt into the lentils, cover, and continue to simmer for another 5 to 10 minutes, until the lentils are tender. Drain the lentils and discard the bay leaf. Place them in a large bowl.

2. Toss the lentils with the vinaigrette, then refrigerate for 20 minutes.

3. Stir in the cucumber, tomatoes, spearmint, and parsley. Before serving, season with salt, freshly ground black pepper, and a squirt of lemon juice.

MIXED RADISH SALAD

SERVES 4, **VEG, GF**

We usually think of radishes as a minor ingredient in mixed salads that provides a watery crunch and sometimes a spicy snap. Here they take center stage along with arugula, basil, and radish sprouts in a lemon–olive oil vinaigrette with Parmesan cheese. If you can't find radish sprouts, substitute sprigs of watercress trimmed of any coarse stems.

1½ pounds mixed radishes, trimmed and sliced

4 cups (about 6 ounces) baby arugula or mixed baby greens

2 cups radish sprouts or watercress

½ cup Basic Lemon Vinaigrette (page 267)

½ cup shaved or grated Parmesan cheese

1. Place the radishes, arugula, and radish sprouts in a large bowl and toss with about ⅓ cup of the dressing. Taste and add more dressing, if needed.

2. To serve, divide the salad among 4 plates and top with Parmesan cheese.

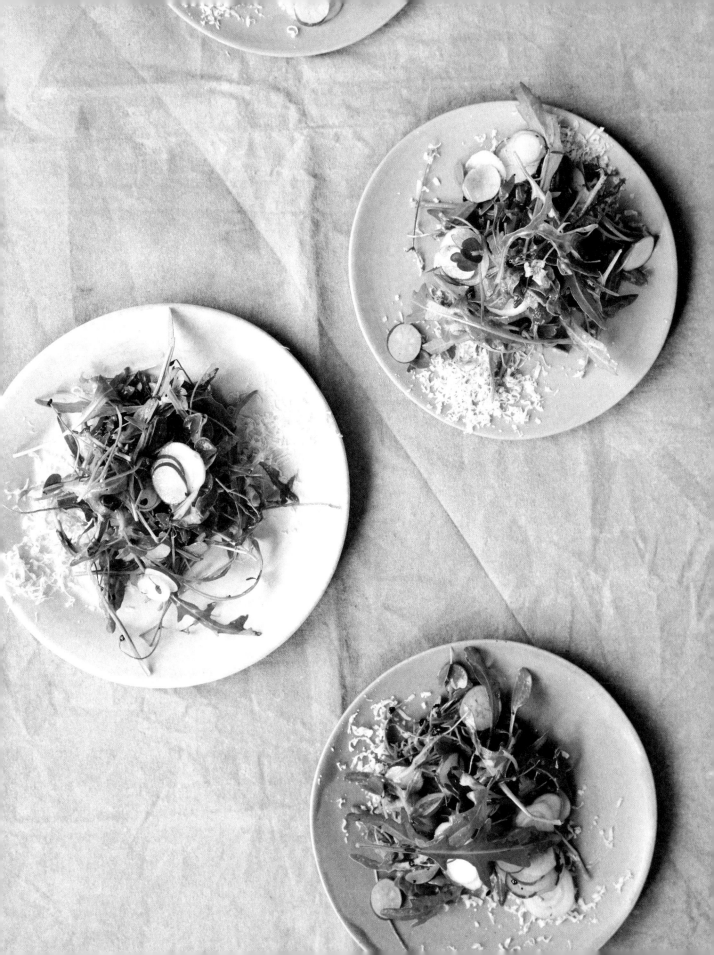

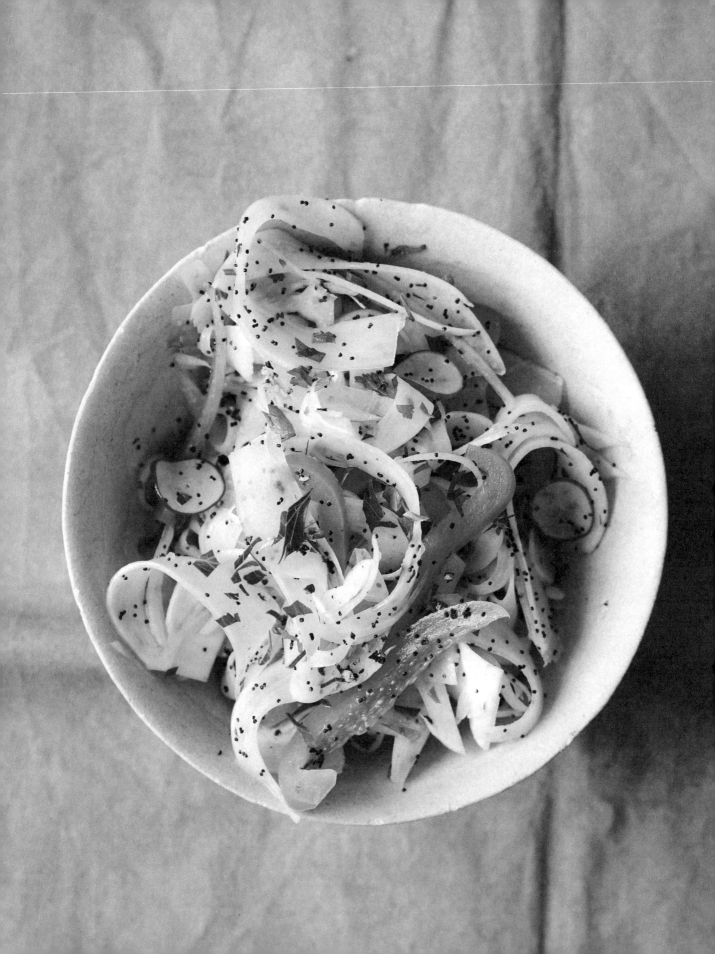

LEMONY FENNEL SLAW

SERVES 4, **V, GF**

A surprising mix of flavors balances the licorice taste of raw fennel. Orange bell pepper, red radishes, and chopped parsley make for a colorful, crunchy slaw.

1 tablespoon poppy seeds

2 large bulbs fennel, thinly shaved, about 2 pounds

1 orange bell pepper, seeded and thinly sliced

3 radishes, cut into thin half-moons

2 tablespoons roughly chopped fresh flat-leaf parsley leaves

1 shallot, thinly sliced

½ cup **Basic Lemon Vinaigrette** (page 267)

1. In a small skillet over medium heat, toast the poppy seeds until fragrant, about 1 to 2 minutes. Stir or shake the pan often.

2. In a large mixing bowl, combine the fennel, bell pepper, radishes, parsley, and shallot. Add as much or as little dressing as you like and mix to combine. Top with toasted poppy seeds and serve.

MOROCCAN ORANGE SALAD
with BLACK OLIVES

SERVES 4, **V, GF**

Orange salads with raw onion and black olives, dressed with olive oil, salt, and pepper, are unfamiliar to North Americans but are common throughout the Mediterranean region, especially in Italy, Spain, and North Africa. They are beautiful and delicious as well as easy to prepare. To "supreme" an orange is to remove its sections without any adhering membrane. You cut off the top and bottom of the orange with a sharp knife, stand it on end, and remove the peel in strips—both the colored zest and underlying white pith—by cutting from top to bottom, following the curve of the fruit. You then cut the sections away from the membrane one by one. (Look up "How to Supreme an Orange" on YouTube for a demonstration.) Use shiny black, oil-cured olives in this dish. Briefly soaking the onion in ice water tones down some of its bite.

½ red onion, thinly sliced across the grain

3 large navel oranges

1 cup pitted oil-cured black olives

1 small garlic clove, pressed and allowed to sit for 10 minutes

3 tablespoons extra-virgin olive oil

¾ teaspoon sweet paprika

½ teaspoon sea salt, plus more to taste

½ teaspoon ground cumin

⅛ teaspoon cayenne pepper

3 tablespoons chopped fresh flat-leaf parsley leaves

1. Place the onion slices in a bowl of ice water and let soak for 10 minutes. Drain, pat dry with paper towels, and set aside.

2. Peel the oranges and supreme them over a large bowl. Once all the sections have been removed and placed in the bowl, squeeze the inner pith and membranes to catch any remaining juice. Add the onions and olives.

3. In a separate bowl, whisk together the remaining ingredients and pour dressing over the salad. Gently toss to ensure all the pieces are evenly coated with dressing, and serve.

RADICCHIO and FRESH PEA SALAD

SERVES 4, **VEG, GF**

This colorful salad is simplicity itself—a perfect balance of texture and flavor.

1 teaspoon plus a pinch of sea salt

1½ cups fresh or frozen peas

3 tablespoons lemon juice

¼ teaspoon freshly ground black pepper

¼ cup extra-virgin olive oil

4 cups (about 6 ounces) baby arugula

1 small radicchio, finely sliced

1 Belgian endive, sliced

½ cup shaved Parmesan cheese

1. In a small pot of boiling water with ½ teaspoon of the salt, blanch fresh peas for 3 minutes or frozen peas for 1 minute. Drain in a colander and rinse with cold water. Set aside.

2. Combine the lemon juice, ½ teaspoon of the salt, and the black pepper in a large salad bowl. Whisk together and then slowly whisk in the oil.

3. Add the peas, arugula, radicchio, endive, and a pinch of salt and toss until well coated. Divide among 4 salad plates and top with shaved Parmesan cheese.

SALMON NIÇOISE with OLIVE, SPEARMINT, and CAPER VINAIGRETTE

SERVES 4, **GF**

Classic salade Niçoise (salad in the style of the French city of Nice, on the Mediterranean coast) consists of tuna, green beans, potatoes, hard-boiled eggs, and, usually, anchovies and the tiny black olives of the region, all in a classic vinaigrette. Here fresh salmon fillet takes the place of tuna—as always, take care not to overcook it—and the anchovies and olives are in the dressing together with spearmint and capers. This is a main-course salad, perfect for a summer lunch.

VINAIGRETTE

¼ cup lemon juice

1 tablespoon minced shallot

2 teaspoons capers, rinsed and roughly chopped

1 teaspoon Dijon mustard

1 finely chopped anchovy (optional)

¼ teaspoon sea salt

⅛ teaspoon freshly ground black pepper

¼ cup extra-virgin olive oil

¼ cup pitted Kalamata olives, chopped

2 tablespoons finely chopped fresh spearmint

SALAD

¾ pound small purple potatoes or French fingerlings, scrubbed

1¼ teaspoons sea salt

2 teaspoons extra-virgin olive oil

2 teaspoons grated lemon zest

2 teaspoons Dijon mustard

1 pound skinless salmon fillet, pinbones removed

Freshly ground black pepper

¾ pound green beans, trimmed

1 cup cherry tomatoes, halved

6 cups (about 8 ounces) salad greens

2 hard-boiled eggs, quartered

12 Niçoise or Kalamata olives

¼ cup roughly chopped fresh basil

4 lemon wedges

1. Preheat the oven to 400°F and line a rimmed baking sheet with parchment paper.

2. To make the dressing, put the lemon juice, shallot, capers, Dijon mustard, anchovy (if desired), salt, and pepper in a small bowl and stir to combine. Slowly pour in the olive oil, whisking all the while, and continue whisking

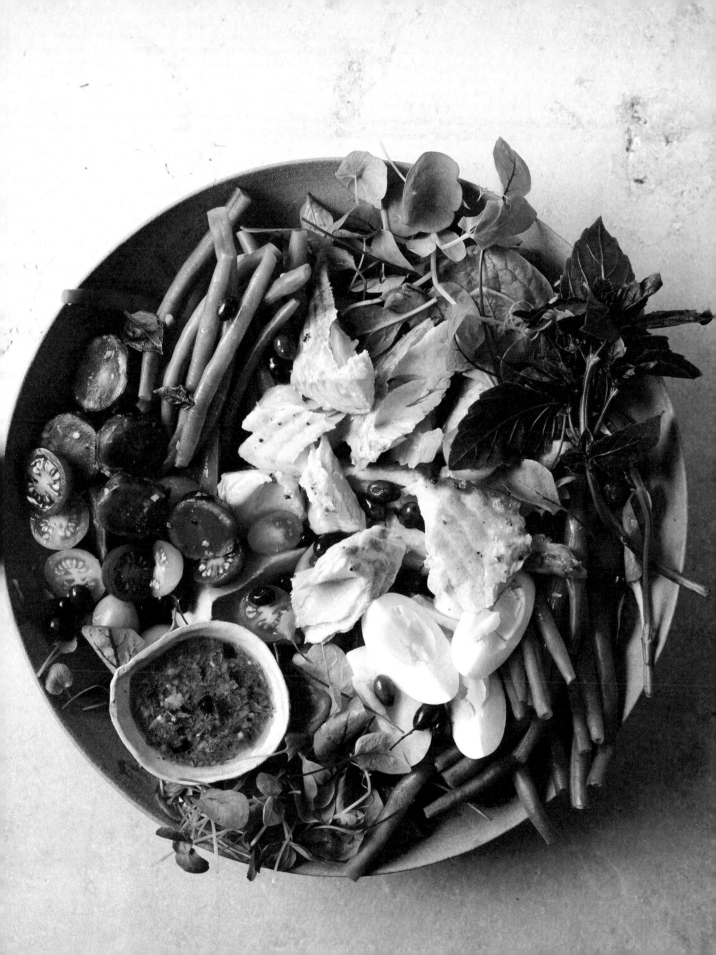

until smooth. Stir in the olives and spearmint. Alternatively, you can blend all the ingredients except the olives and spearmint in a jar with the solid disk of an immersion blender, then stir in the olives and spearmint.

3. In a 4-quart pot, cover the potatoes with cold water and 1 teaspoon of the salt. Bring the water to a boil, then reduce the heat and simmer, uncovered, until potatoes are just tender, about 10 minutes.

4. While the potatoes cook, place the olive oil, lemon zest, and mustard in a small bowl and stir to combine. Place the salmon on the baking sheet and spread the mixture evenly over both sides of the fish, then season it with the remaining ¼ teaspoon salt and freshly ground pepper.

5. Roast until just opaque but still slightly translucent in the center, about 7 to 9 minutes. Break the salmon into pieces.

6. Transfer the potatoes with a slotted spoon to a bowl. Add the green beans to the boiling water and cook, uncovered, until crisp-tender, about 4 to 5 minutes. Drain and transfer to an ice bath to stop the cooking.

7. Halve the potatoes while still warm and toss with 2 tablespoons of the dressing.

8. Toss the green beans and cherry tomatoes with a tablespoon of the dressing. In a different bowl, toss the greens with enough dressing to coat. Divide the greens among 4 plates, then add the potatoes, tomatoes, green beans, salmon, eggs, and olives. Sprinkle with basil. Serve with lemon wedges and the remaining dressing on the side.

SHREDDED BRUSSELS SPROUTS
with LEMON-CAPER DRESSING

SERVES 4, **V, GF**

This is a novel take on coleslaw: raw, shredded Brussels sprouts and red cabbage in a zesty vinaigrette. It's fresh, colorful, tasty, and full of beneficial phytonutrients.

DRESSING

¼ cup lemon juice

2 teaspoons grated lemon zest

1 large shallot, finely chopped

2 teaspoons Dijon mustard

2 tablespoons capers, rinsed, drained, and chopped

½ teaspoon sea salt

¼ teaspoon freshly ground black pepper

¼ cup extra-virgin olive oil

SALAD

½ pound Brussels sprouts, trimmed and finely shredded

¼ head red cabbage, shredded

½ cup raw almonds, toasted and chopped (page 274)

1. In a bowl, whisk together all the dressing ingredients except the oil. Whisk in the oil in a steady stream. Alternatively, you can blend all the dressing ingredients together in a jar with the solid disk of an immersion blender.

2. In a large bowl, combine the Brussels sprouts and cabbage and pour half of the dressing around the sides of the bowl. Gently toss the vegetables until all are well coated with the dressing. Add more dressing to taste.

3. To serve, divide among 4 salad plates and top with the almonds.

CABBAGE SLAW with GINGER-CURRY VINAIGRETTE and TOASTED CASHEWS

SERVES 6, **V**, **GF**

The curry vinaigrette and toasted cashews make this anything but a typical slaw. It's colorful and texturally interesting, and it will surprise you with its bold mix of flavors.

SALAD

½ small head red cabbage, thinly sliced (about 2 cups)

½ small head Napa or green cabbage, thinly sliced (about 2 cups)

1 large carrot, peeled and cut into matchsticks

1 green apple, peeled, cored, and cut into matchsticks

¼ cup chopped fresh cilantro

¼ cup chopped fresh spearmint

¼ cup raisins

½ cup raw cashews, toasted (page 274)

VINAIGRETTE

2 tablespoons lime juice

1½ teaspoons peeled grated ginger

1 tablespoon unseasoned rice vinegar

1 tablespoon grade B maple syrup

½ teaspoon sea salt

½ teaspoon curry powder

⅓ cup extra-virgin olive oil

1. Combine the vegetables, apple, herbs, and raisins in a large bowl. Reserve the cashews to garnish the finished salad.

2. Whisk the dressing ingredients together, pour over the salad, and toss to combine. Top with toasted cashews.

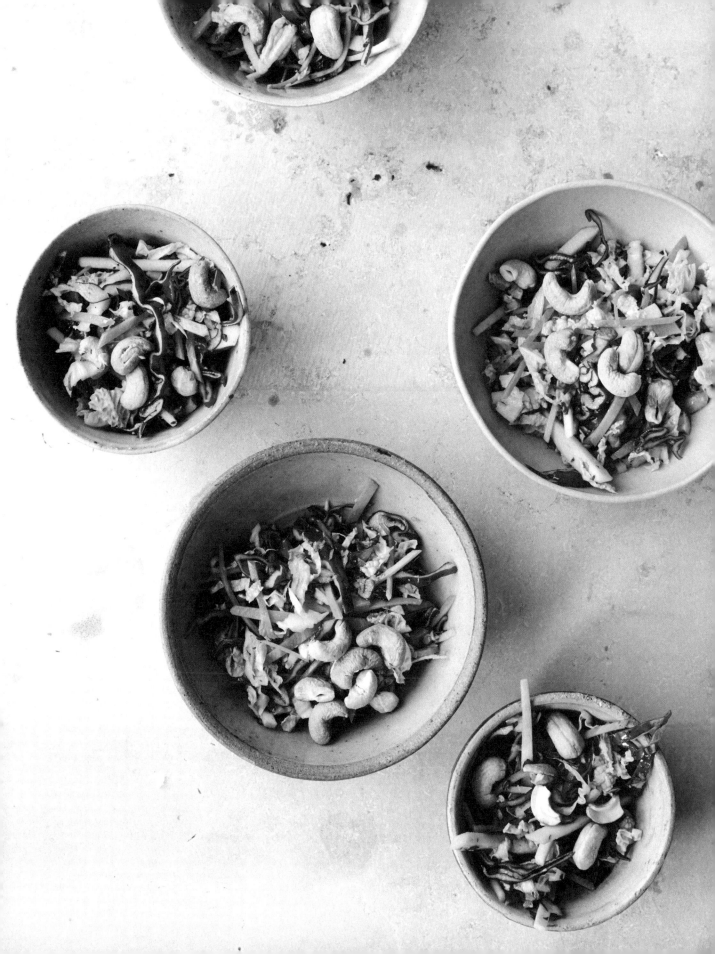

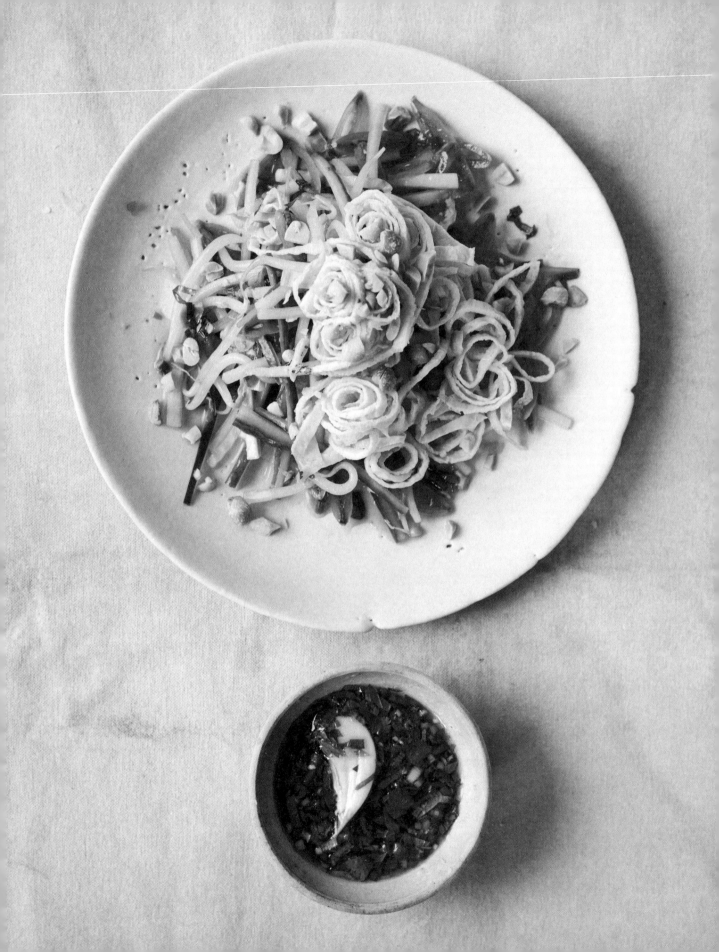

THAI EGG SALAD
with SUGAR SNAP PEAS

SERVES 4, **GF**

Not like any egg salad you've ever tasted. Thin, plain "omelets" are shredded and placed atop a mound of chilled, sliced raw vegetables dressed with a vibrant mixture of flavors characteristic of Thai cuisine: basil, spearmint, cilantro, chili, garlic, fish sauce, lime juice, and sugar—with chopped nuts as a garnish. Colorful and fresh, novel and delicious, this salad makes a satisfying one-dish meal. A lot of slicing and chopping, but the result is worth it.

SALAD

2 English cucumbers, peeled and thinly sliced

1½ cups sugar snap peas, cut on the bias into ½-inch slices

2 carrots, peeled and julienned

½ cup tightly packed fresh spearmint leaves, sliced

½ cup tightly packed fresh basil leaves, sliced

½ cup tightly packed fresh cilantro leaves, roughly chopped

1 cup bean sprouts

4 large eggs

4 teaspoons grapeseed oil

3 scallions, white and light green parts, thinly sliced on the bias

¼ cup chopped dry-roasted unsalted peanuts or cashews

DRESSING

2 garlic cloves, pressed and allowed to sit for 10 minutes

3 tablespoons fish sauce

¼ cup lime juice

1 tablespoon evaporated cane sugar

Pinch of cayenne pepper, to taste

¼ cup grapeseed oil

1. In a large bowl, combine the cucumbers, snap peas, carrots, spearmint, basil, and cilantro. Place in the refrigerator to chill.

2. Bring a small pot of water to a boil and blanch the sprouts for 30 seconds. Drain, plunge in cold water, drain again, and dry with paper or kitchen towel. Add sprouts to the rest of the vegetables in the refrigerator.

3. Whisk together the dressing ingredients and let stand on the counter.

4. Crack the eggs into a bowl and whisk them well. Heat 1 teaspoon of the grapeseed oil in a large nonstick pan over medium heat and pour in ¼ of the egg mixture. Tilt the pan to spread the egg into a thin circle and cook for 1 to 2 minutes or until fully set. Use a spatula to remove the egg and lay it flat on a plate. Repeat with the remaining oil and eggs. Once all are cooked, roll up the egg circles into cigars and thinly shred them.

5. Pour the dressing over the chilled vegetables and gently toss. Divide among 4 plates and top with the eggs, scallions, and nuts.

MEXICAN SALAD

SERVES 4 TO 6, **VEG**

There is a lot of texture in this southwestern-style salad. The combination of romaine, tomatoes, radishes, black beans, creamy avocado, baked tortillas, and toasted pumpkin seeds, all coated in a tangy lime vinaigrette, makes this dish a crunch-lover's dream.

2 corn tortillas

DRESSING

2 tablespoons lime juice

2 tablespoons extra-virgin olive oil

½ teaspoon sea salt

⅛ to ¼ teaspoon cayenne pepper

1 avocado

SALAD

4 romaine lettuce hearts, trimmed, leaves separated and roughly torn

12 cherry tomatoes, halved

6 radishes, quartered

½ cup roughly chopped cilantro leaves

1 avocado, cut into chunks

1 (15-ounce) can black beans, rinsed, drained, and spritzed with lime

2 tablespoons raw pumpkin seeds, toasted (page 274)

2 tablespoons queso fresco, crumbled

1. Preheat the oven to 350°F and line a rimmed baking sheet with parchment paper.

2. Place the tortillas on the baking sheet and bake for 10 minutes or until crispy. Remove from the oven and allow to cool. When they are cool to the touch, break them into bite-size pieces and set aside.

3. Place the dressing ingredients with ¼ cup of water in a blender or blend in a jar with the solid disk of an immersion blender until smooth.

4. Toss the lettuce with 6 tablespoons of dressing. Add tomatoes, radishes, cilantro, avocado, black beans, pumpkin seeds, and tortillas. Divide among 4 to 6 plates and top each portion with some queso fresco. (Store remaining dressing in a jar in the refrigerator for up to 2 days.)

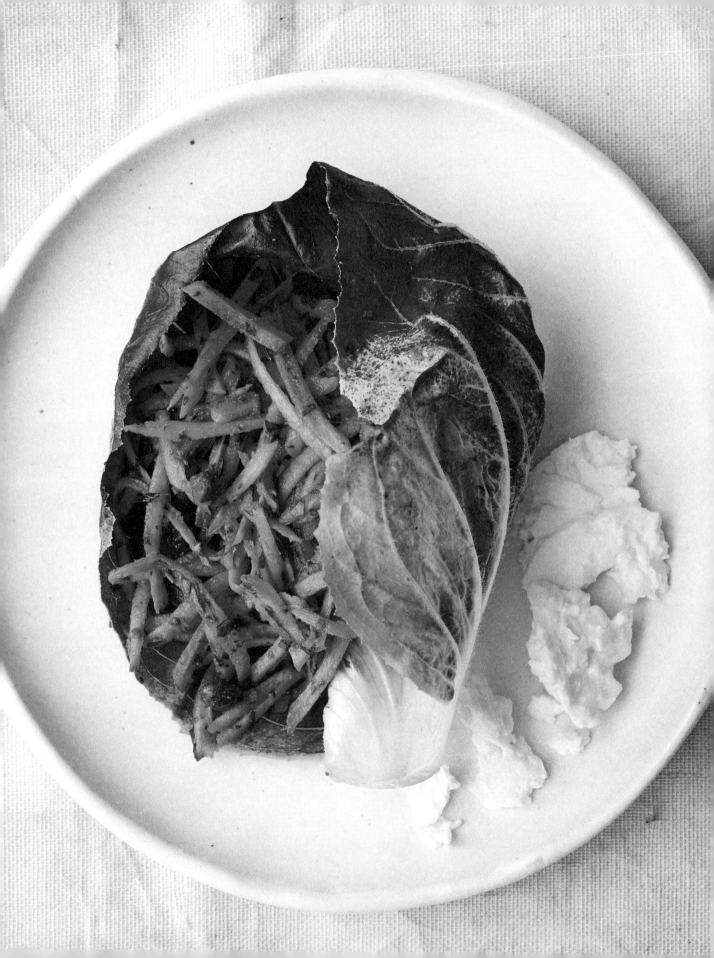

TUNISIAN SPICED CARROT SALAD

SERVES 4 TO 6, **VEG**, **V***, **GF**

A great way to enjoy raw carrots. The blend of spices and herbs in the dressing gives them a real kick. This can be a starter, a salad, or a side dish. However you make use of it, it will give you a big helping of protective phytonutrients in addition to delighting your senses.

2 tablespoons extra-virgin olive oil

2 garlic cloves, pressed and allowed to sit for 10 minutes

1 teaspoon caraway seeds

½ teaspoon ground cumin

¾ teaspoon paprika

2 tablespoons lemon juice, or more to taste

½ teaspoon sea salt, or more to taste

1 pound carrots, peeled and coarsely shredded with grater or food processor

3 tablespoons minced fresh flat-leaf parsley leaves

3 tablespoons minced fresh spearmint

1 tablespoon capers, plus a little caper brine

Butterhead lettuce or radicchio (optional)

4 ounces crumbled feta (optional)

1. Heat the olive oil in a small skillet over medium heat. Sauté the garlic, caraway, cumin, and paprika until fragrant, about 2 minutes. Remove from the heat, add lemon juice and salt, and add the mixture to the shredded carrots in a bowl. Add the parsley, spearmint, capers, and a little caper brine. Mix well. Taste and adjust with more lemon juice or salt, if necessary.

2. Serve the salad on leaves of butterhead lettuce or radicchio, if desired, or divide among 4 to 6 plates and top each portion with feta cheese.

WARM MUSHROOM SALAD

SERVES 4, **VEG, GF**

Sautéed mushrooms flavored with herbs on a bed of radicchio or cool greens tossed with a lemon-mustard vinaigrette make a substantial salad that can be the centerpiece of a light meal.

1 tablespoon extra-virgin olive oil

2 pounds mixed mushrooms (shiitake, oyster, cremini, or wild), thickly sliced

2 teaspoons finely chopped fresh thyme or ¼ teaspoon dried thyme

1 teaspoon finely chopped fresh rosemary or ⅛ teaspoon dried rosemary

¼ teaspoon sea salt

6 cups (about 8 ounces) radicchio or mixed greens

1 cup Basic Lemon Vinaigrette (page 267)

½ cup shaved pecorino or Parmesan cheese (optional)

1. Heat the olive oil in a large skillet over medium-high heat. Add the mushrooms, thyme, rosemary, and salt and sauté for 8 to 10 minutes or until brown.

2. Lightly dress the greens with the vinaigrette and arrange them on a serving platter. Spoon the mushrooms on top of the radicchio or greens and top with shaved cheese and more of the dressing.

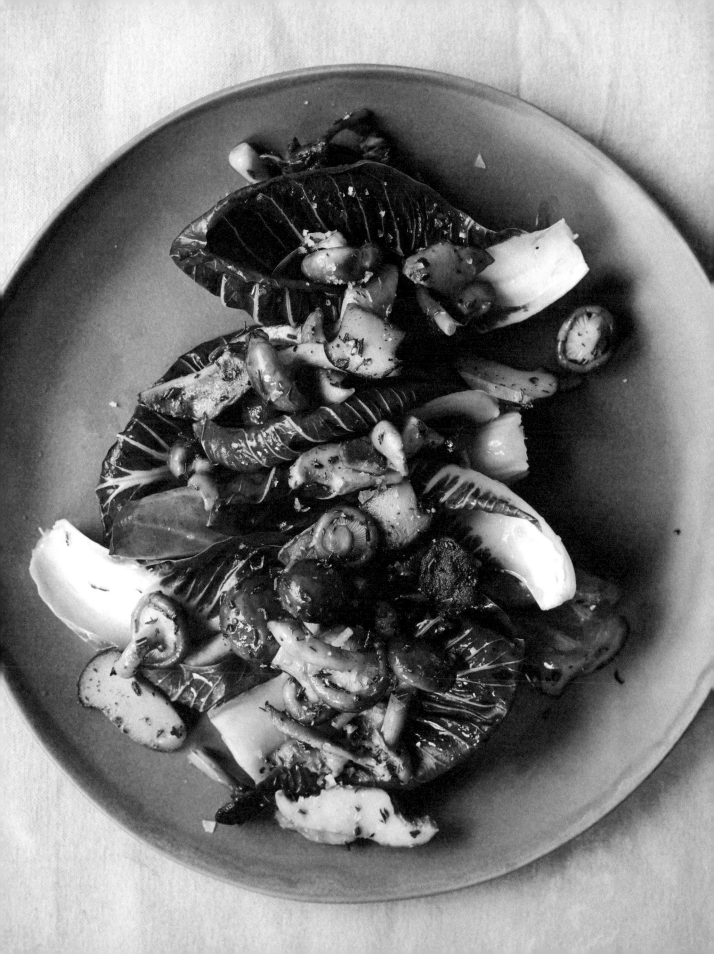

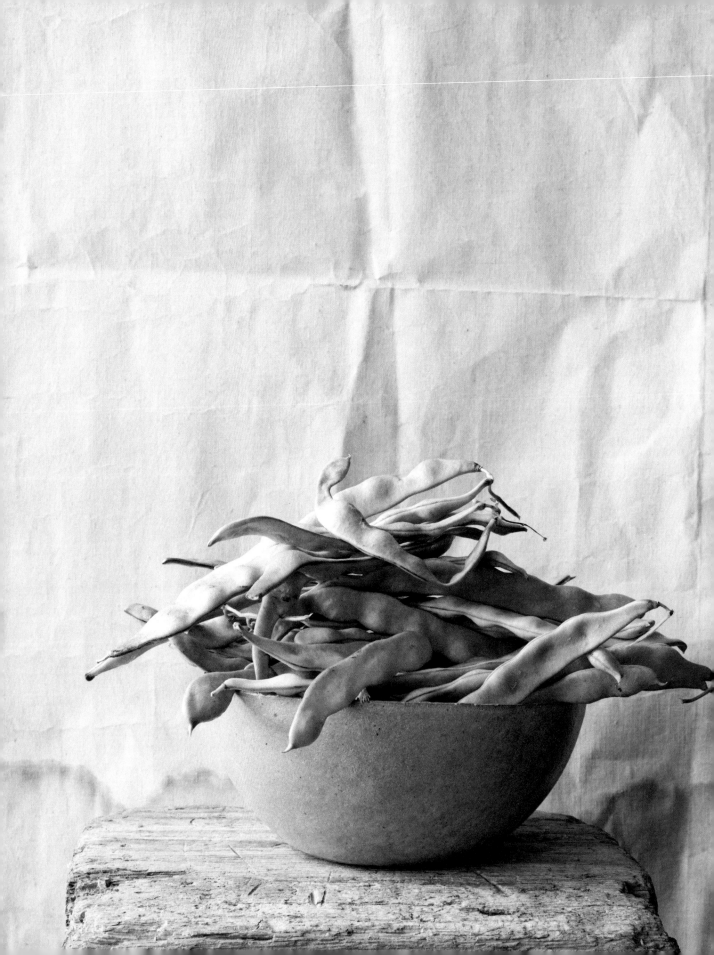

Vegetables

We're always told to eat more fruits and vegetables. I think we should concentrate on vegetables, because they are the best sources of micronutrients, fiber, and protective phytonutrients and don't have the sugar content of fruit. Many of the beneficial compounds in vegetables are pigments, with each hue having different properties. I recommend eating across the color spectrum—every day if possible—from white-green to yellow to orange, red, and purple. So many people I know say they do not have the time or know-how to cook fresh vegetables; others tell me they just don't like them. It took me a while to learn to like some—beets, Brussels sprouts, even broccoli—because growing up, I had them only overcooked or ruined in other ways. Preparing vegetables for optimum taste can be easy and quick. Broccoli, for instance, is best after just a few minutes of steaming so that it comes out bright green and crisp-tender. The recipes that follow will introduce you to easy and appealing preparations of some of my favorite roots, tubers, leaves, and stalks, as well as to the immature fruits that we think of as vegetables, like green beans, snap peas, cucumbers, and zucchini. I hope they will help you bring more vegetables to your table.

Recipes marked **veg** are vegetarian, those marked **v** are vegan, and those marked **gf** are gluten-free. The symbols **veg***, **v***, and **gf*** indicate recipes that can be modified to be vegetarian, vegan, or gluten-free by substituting or omitting specific ingredients.

BOLD GARLICKY DARK LEAFY GREENS

SERVES 4, **VEG, V*, GF***

I do not get the custom of cooking greens to death. To my taste, they are most appealing when sautéed quickly until just tender. Here, lemon zest and juice and a touch of maple syrup balance the slight bitterness of the greens. Garlic, red pepper flakes, and shaved Parmesan make this dish even more delicious.

2 tablespoons extra-virgin olive oil

1 red onion, cut into half-moons

¼ teaspoon plus a pinch of sea salt

2 garlic cloves, pressed and allowed to sit for 10 minutes

Generous pinch of crushed red pepper flakes

1 large bunch black (Tuscan or lacinato) kale or Swiss chard, stemmed and chopped into bite-size pieces

1½ teaspoons grated lemon zest

1 tablespoon lemon juice

1 teaspoon grade B maple syrup

1 tablespoon whole-grain toasted bread crumbs, or 1 tablespoon chopped toasted almonds

2 tablespoons shaved Parmesan cheese

1. Heat the olive oil in a large, deep skillet over medium-high heat. Add the onions and a pinch of salt and sauté for 3 minutes. Decrease the heat to medium-low and cook, stirring occasionally, until the onions are slightly golden, about 5 minutes.

2. Increase the heat to medium. Add the garlic and red pepper flakes and sauté until the garlic is lightly golden, about 20 seconds. Add the kale to the skillet along with another pinch of salt and sauté until bright green and wilted, about 3 minutes. Add a tablespoon of water, cover, and cook until just tender, no more than 4 minutes more.

3. Stir in the lemon zest, lemon juice, and maple syrup. Divide the greens among 4 serving plates and top with the bread crumbs and shavings of Parmesan.

BROCCOLI with WASABI BUTTER or MISO BUTTER

SERVES 4, **VEG**, **GF**

This is a twist on plain old steamed broccoli, which too often is tasteless. The miso is the salt component in the miso butter. If you choose to use wasabi butter, you may need to add a pinch of sea salt to this dish.

1¼ pounds broccoli, broken into florets, stems peeled and cut into chunks

1 to 2 tablespoons Wasabi Butter (page 271) or Miso Butter (page 270)

1. Using a steamer basket over an inch or two of lightly boiling water, steam the broccoli for 4 to 5 minutes until it's bright green and just crisp-tender.

2. Place into a serving bowl and dollop the Wasabi Butter or Miso Butter on the broccoli. Toss to coat and serve.

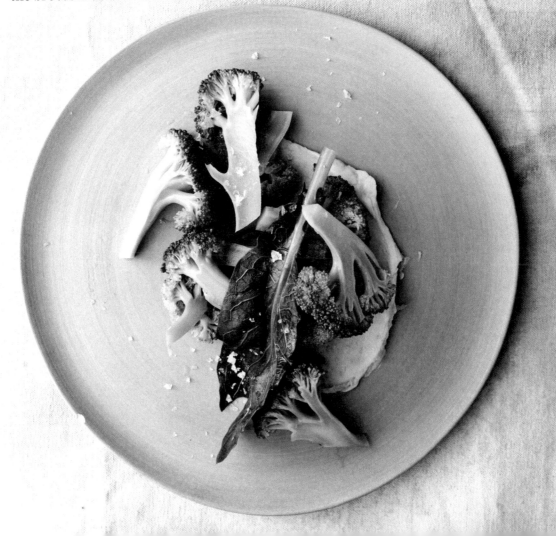

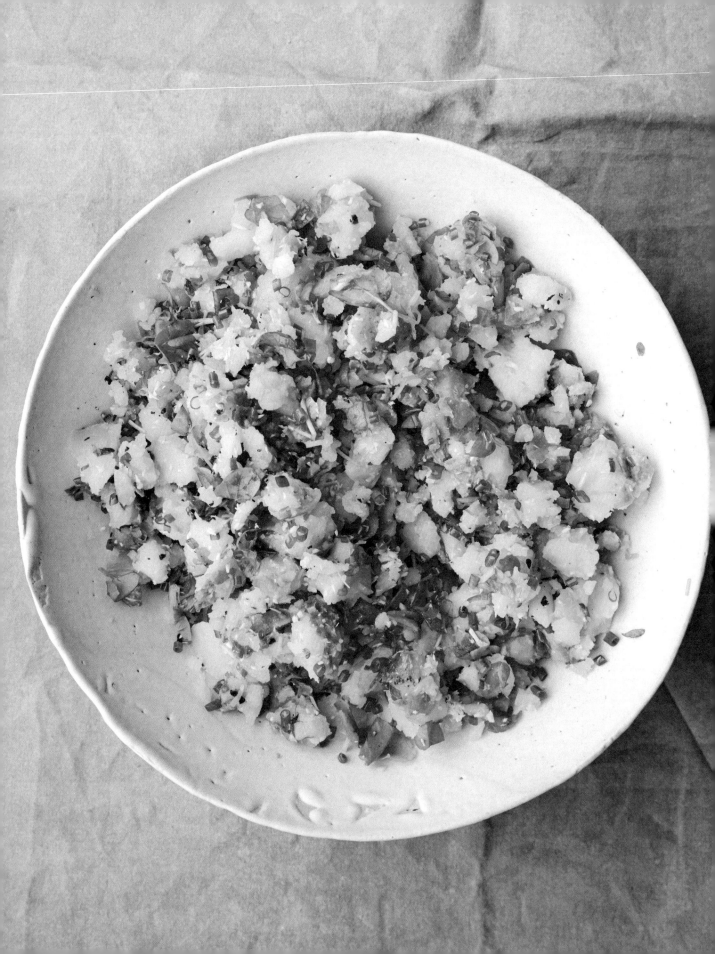

SMASHED POTATOES with HORSERADISH, GREENS, and HERBS

SERVES 6, **V, GF**

Roughly smashed potatoes flavored with olive oil and fresh horseradish and mixed with chopped raw greens are a revelation, better than any butter- and cream-laden mashed potatoes you've ever had. If you can't find red-skinned French fingerlings, look for other new or small boiling potatoes, preferably organic. The texture of this dish should be chunky and rustic, far from a smooth puree.

1½ pounds red fingerling potatoes, scrubbed

1½ teaspoons sea salt

3 tablespoons extra-virgin olive oil, plus more for finishing

3 tablespoons Prepared Fresh Horseradish (page 268), or more to taste

Freshly ground black pepper

2 tablespoons chopped fresh chives

1 cup roughly chopped watercress or arugula, coarse stems removed

1. Place the potatoes in a medium pot and cover with cold water and 1 teaspoon of the salt. Bring the water to a boil and cook until the potatoes are just tender, about 10 minutes or until you can slide the tip of a knife all the way through without resistance.

2. Drain the potatoes and return them to the pot. Add the remaining ½ teaspoon salt and the olive oil, then smash the potatoes with a potato masher or the back of a fork.

3. Stir in the horseradish, some freshly ground black pepper, and chives. Fold in the roughly chopped greens, transfer the potatoes to a serving bowl, and drizzle some olive oil on top.

GREEN BEANS in TOMATO SAUCE

SERVES 4, V, GF

I prefer flat Romano beans for this typical Mediterranean dish, which I make frequently in midsummer, when I'm inundated with beans from my garden in British Columbia. If tomatoes are ready at the same time, I'll use them (peeled and seeded) for the sauce, along with fresh herbs. But this quick version with canned tomatoes and dried herbs is almost as good. As usual with vegetable recipes in this book, it is important not to overcook the beans. The difference between crunchy-tender perfection and all-the-way-through softness is only a minute or two. Please try a bean a short time before you think they might be done.

3 tablespoons extra-virgin olive oil

1 onion, sliced

½ to 1 teaspoon crushed red pepper flakes (optional)

1 (15-ounce) can peeled and crushed Italian tomatoes, with juice

2 garlic cloves, pressed and allowed to sit for 10 minutes

1 teaspoon evaporated cane sugar

1 teaspoon dried oregano

1 tablespoon dried basil

Pinch of ground allspice

½ teaspoon sea salt, or more to taste

1 pound Romano beans or other green beans, trimmed and cut into 2-inch pieces

1. Heat the oil in a skillet over medium heat, add the onion, and cook, stirring frequently, until the onion is translucent, about 4 minutes. Add the red pepper flakes and tomatoes. Add the remaining ingredients except for the beans, bring to a boil, then reduce the heat and allow to simmer until the sauce is thickened, about 10 minutes. Taste and adjust with salt or red pepper flakes, if necessary.

2. Add the beans to the skillet and mix well. Cover and allow the beans to cook until they are just tender, about 5 to 7 minutes. If the mixture is too dry, add a little water to prevent it from sticking to the pan—not too much, because the sauce should be thick. When the beans are just tender, uncover and cook 1 minute more.

3. Serve hot, at room temperature, or chilled.

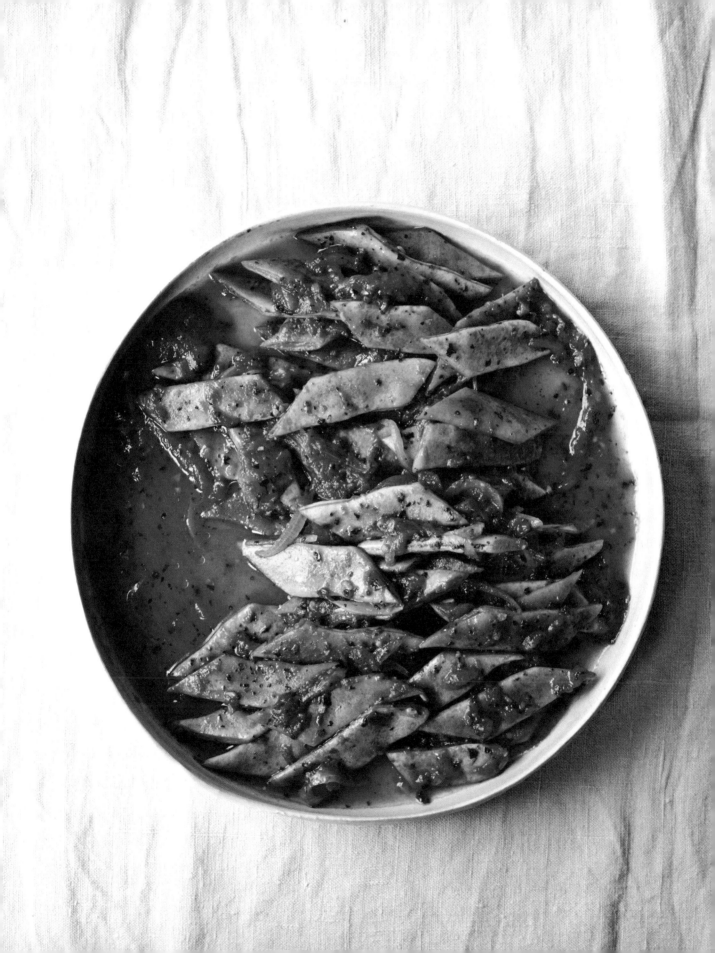

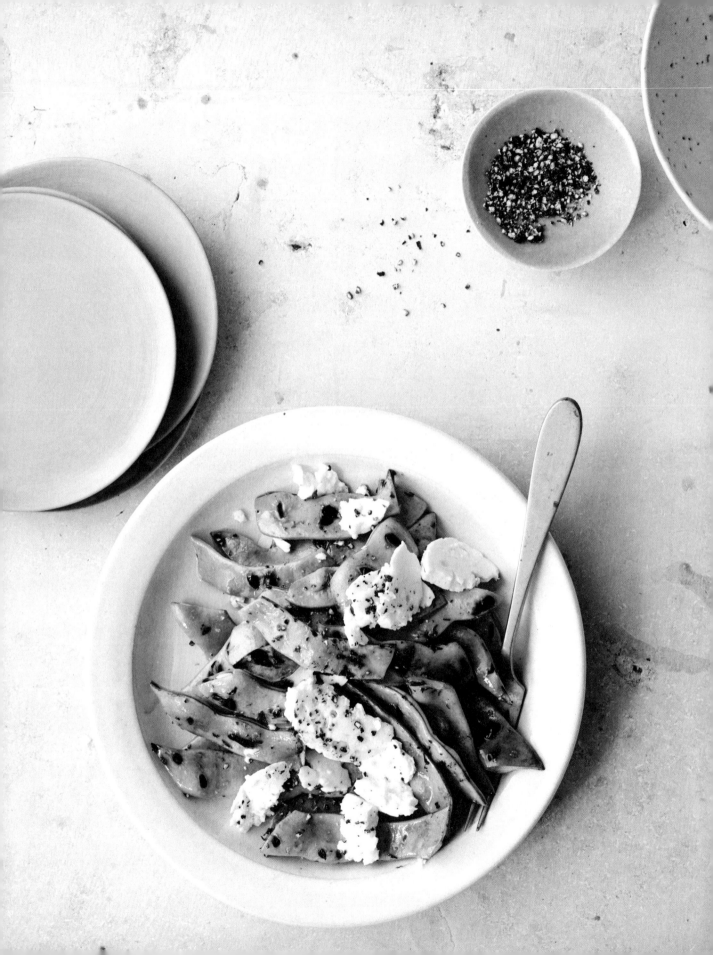

GRILLED ROMANO BEANS

SERVES 4, **VEG**, **V***, **GF**

Grilled green beans? Yes! You will be delighted by this quick and unusual preparation. Feel free to play with flavors and garnishes. Serve the beans immediately; they should be warm and still a bit crunchy. For variations, try replacing the thyme with oregano and the feta with Parmesan. Blue Lake green beans can be substituted for Romanos.

1 pound Romano beans, trimmed

1 tablespoon extra-virgin olive oil

1 tablespoon chopped fresh thyme or 1 teaspoon dried thyme

½ teaspoon sea salt

¼ teaspoon freshly ground black pepper

2 ounces crumbled feta cheese

1. In a large bowl, toss the beans with the olive oil, thyme, salt, and pepper.

2. Place the beans on a hot grill pan or in a grill basket and cook for 2 minutes on each side until just tender with a few grill marks.

3. Place the grilled beans on a serving platter and top with crumbled feta.

PAN-ROASTED JERUSALEM ARTICHOKES with SAGE

SERVES 4, **V, GF**

Jerusalem artichokes are the tubers of a species of sunflower native to eastern North America. Italian immigrants called the plant *girasole*, the Italian term for "sunflower," and English speakers turned that into "Jerusalem." The vegetable is now often labeled "sunchoke" in markets. High in protein and micronutrients and surprisingly low in starch, Jerusalem artichokes should be peeled and quickly cooked. (Raw, unpeeled tubers can cause flatulence and gastrointestinal upset.) Here they are browned in olive oil and flavored with sage for a tasty and unusual side dish.

3 tablespoons extra-virgin olive oil, plus more for finishing

1½ pounds Jerusalem artichokes, peeled and cut into ½-inch slices

Sea salt and freshly ground black pepper, to taste

1 tablespoon finely chopped fresh sage or 1 teaspoon dried sage

4 garlic cloves, pressed and allowed to sit for 10 minutes

⅓ cup dry (white) vermouth

1 teaspoon lemon juice

2 tablespoons finely chopped fresh flat-leaf parsley leaves

1. Heat the oil in a large skillet over medium-high heat. Add the Jerusalem artichokes and cook for a few minutes on each side until golden brown. Season with salt and pepper, and add the sage, garlic, and vermouth. Reduce the heat to medium-low, cover, and cook, stirring occasionally, for 15 to 20 minutes or until fork-tender.

2. Remove the Jerusalem artichokes from the heat and season with lemon juice, salt, and pepper. Drizzle with a bit of olive oil, garnish with parsley, and serve.

PERUVIAN CAULIFLOWER with LIME

SERVES 4, **V, GF**

I had this very simple dish at an excellent floating restaurant in Iquitos, Peru's metropolis on the Amazon. It was cooling and refreshing in the hot, steamy climate of that city. The only caution is not to overcook the cauliflower. Test a piece slightly before you think it's done; it should be just crunchy-tender.

1 large head cauliflower, cut into medium florets

½ cup finely chopped fresh flat-leaf parsley leaves

3 tablespoons finely sliced fresh chives

Juice of 3 limes

½ cup extra-virgin olive oil

¾ teaspoon sea salt

1 teaspoon freshly ground black pepper

1. Using a steamer basket over an inch or two of lightly boiling water, steam the cauliflower until tender but still crunchy, about 5 to 6 minutes. Pour out onto a wide serving dish and allow to cool.

2. Whisk the remaining ingredients together in a large bowl and let the dressing sit for 5 minutes for the flavors to meld.

3. Add the cauliflower to the dressing and thoroughly toss until completely coated. Let sit for at least 5 minutes before returning to the serving plate.

PAN-SEARED CARROTS and KALE with HAZELNUTS

SERVES 4, **V, GF**

Vegetables of all colors seem to look right with lacinato kale. Here, pan-seared carrots tame kale's bitter nature. The toasted hazelnuts add a wonderful surprise to this bright green and orange vegetable sauté that's rich in flavor and nutrients.

3 tablespoons extra-virgin olive oil

¾ pound carrots, peeled and cut on the bias into ¼-inch pieces

2 shallots, cut into ½-inch rings

½ teaspoon grade B maple syrup, or more to taste

Pinch of crushed red pepper flakes

½ teaspoon sea salt, or more to taste

2 bunches black kale, stemmed and torn into bite-size pieces

1 tablespoon lemon juice

1 teaspoon grated lemon zest

⅛ teaspoon ground nutmeg

2 tablespoons toasted and chopped hazelnuts (page 274)

1. In a large sauté pan, heat 2 tablespoons of the olive oil over medium-high heat. Add the carrots, shallots, ¼ teaspoon of the maple syrup, red pepper flakes, and ¼ teaspoon of the salt. Stir and cook for about 5 minutes or until the vegetables are tender and caramelized. Transfer them to a plate.

2. To the same pan, add the remaining 1 tablespoon oil, kale, and the remaining ¼ teaspoon salt. Give a stir and, if necessary, add a tablespoon of water. Sauté until the kale is tender, about 2 minutes.

3. Stir in the lemon juice, zest, the remaining ¼ teaspoon maple syrup, and the nutmeg. Taste and adjust with another pinch of salt or drop of maple syrup if necessary.

4. Add back the shallots and carrots along with the hazelnuts. Toss together and serve immediately.

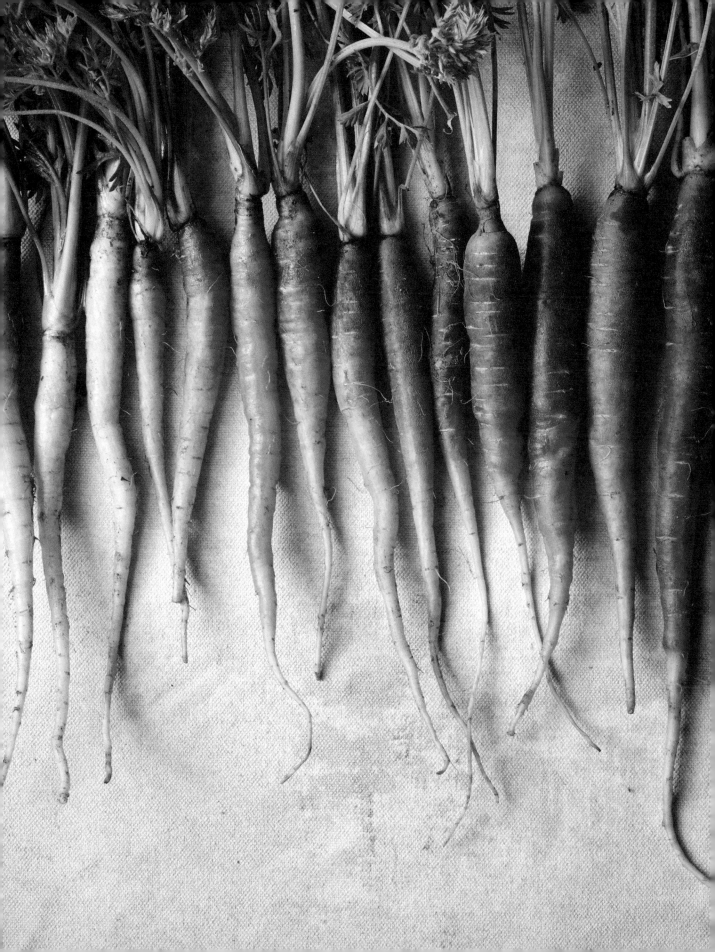

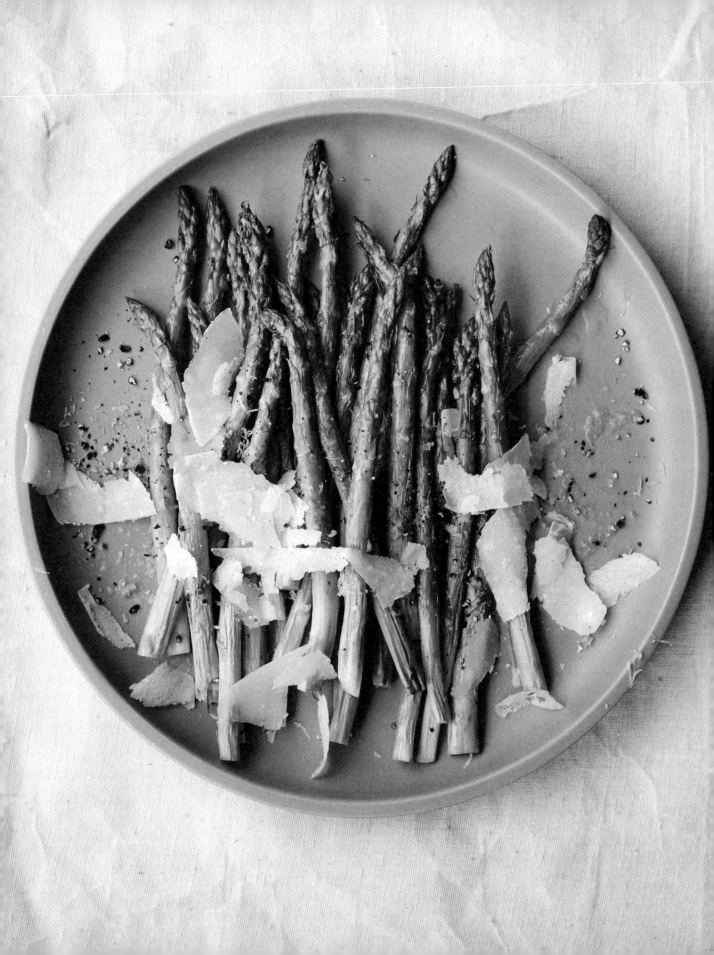

ROASTED ASPARAGUS with LEMON and PARMESAN

SERVES 4, VEG, V*, GF

This is not the overcooked stringy asparagus of the past. Roasting brings out the vegetable's naturally sweet flavor. If you want to go the extra mile, a wise Italian cook taught me to peel away the tough outer layer at the lower end of each stalk to expose the tender flesh beneath. (Use a vegetable peeler for this; it takes just a few extra minutes.)

2 bunches asparagus (about 2 pounds), trimmed

2 teaspoons extra-virgin olive oil

½ teaspoon sea salt

¼ teaspoon freshly ground black pepper

1 teaspoon fresh lemon juice

1 teaspoon grated lemon zest

2 tablespoons freshly shaved Parmesan cheese

1. Preheat the oven to 400°F and line a rimmed baking sheet with parchment paper.

2. Put the asparagus on the baking sheet in a single layer. Drizzle with olive oil and sprinkle with the salt and pepper. Toss gently to evenly coat the asparagus. Bake for 8 minutes or until just barely tender.

3. Toss the asparagus with the lemon juice and lemon zest. Transfer it to a platter and sprinkle with freshly shaved Parmesan cheese.

ROASTED CARROTS with DUKKAH

SERVES 4, **V, GF**

Here, everyday carrots get a quick makeover in the oven. They're roasted until golden and sweet, then sprinkled with dukkah, a Middle Eastern spice blend that makes them exotic and irresistible.

4 large carrots, cut on the bias into 2-inch pieces

1½ tablespoons extra-virgin olive oil

½ teaspoon sea salt

2 teaspoons Dukkah (page 273)

1. Preheat the oven to 425°F and line a rimmed baking sheet with parchment paper.

2. In a large bowl, toss the carrots with the olive oil and salt.

3. Spread the carrots in one layer on the baking sheet. Roast in the oven for 15 minutes or until tender and golden. Sprinkle with the Dukkah and serve hot.

SPICED ROASTED KABOCHA SQUASH

SERVES 6, **V, GF**

Kabocha, or Japanese pumpkin, is a sweet, orange-fleshed winter squash with a fine texture when baked. It has a hard shell and a center filled with seeds. To cut it, insert a heavy knife into the center so that the squash lifts with the knife. With the palm of your hand on the dull side of the blade, lift and tap the squash on your cutting board a few times until it cracks open. You can then easily slice it in half. If you can't find a kabocha, use a butternut squash.

2 tablespoons extra-virgin olive oil

½ teaspoon sea salt, plus more to taste

¼ teaspoon ground allspice

¼ teaspoon crushed red pepper flakes

¼ teaspoon ground cinnamon

2½ to 3 pounds kabocha squash, peeled, seeded, and cut into 1-inch slices (half-moons)

1. Preheat the oven to 475°F and line a rimmed baking sheet with parchment paper.

2. In a small bowl, combine the olive oil, salt, allspice, red pepper flakes, and cinnamon.

3. Put the squash on the baking sheet and drizzle with the olive oil mixture. Toss with your hands to coat, then spread the squash out in a single layer. Sprinkle with a couple more pinches of salt.

4. Roast in the oven for about 15 to 20 minutes or until tender. Transfer the squash to a platter. Serve hot or at room temperature.

ROASTED CAULIFLOWER

SERVES 4, **VEG, GF***

So simple, quick, and good, this is one of my favorite ways to prepare cauliflower. I always try a piece at 13 minutes to make sure I don't cook the cauliflower past the point of delicious crunchy tenderness. Bread crumbs add a nice textural contrast but can be left out if you prefer. I usually add a bit of the caper juice for extra flavor. This is a crowd-pleaser, even for those who normally disdain cauliflower.

1 pound cauliflower, cut into bite-size florets

4 garlic cloves, pressed and allowed to sit for 10 minutes

3 tablespoons extra-virgin olive oil, or more if necessary

Sea salt and crushed red pepper flakes, to taste

¼ cup bread crumbs (page 274)

½ cup freshly grated Parmesan cheese

⅛ teaspoon ground nutmeg

¼ cup chopped fresh flat-leaf parsley leaves

1. Preheat the oven to 375°F and line a rimmed baking sheet with parchment paper.

2. In a bowl, mix the cauliflower, garlic, and olive oil. If necessary, add a little more olive oil to evenly coat the cauliflower. Add the bread crumbs, Parmesan cheese, and nutmeg and mix well.

3. Spread the cauliflower mixture evenly on a baking sheet. Roast until just tender and very lightly browned, about 13 to 15 minutes. Sprinkle with parsley and serve hot.

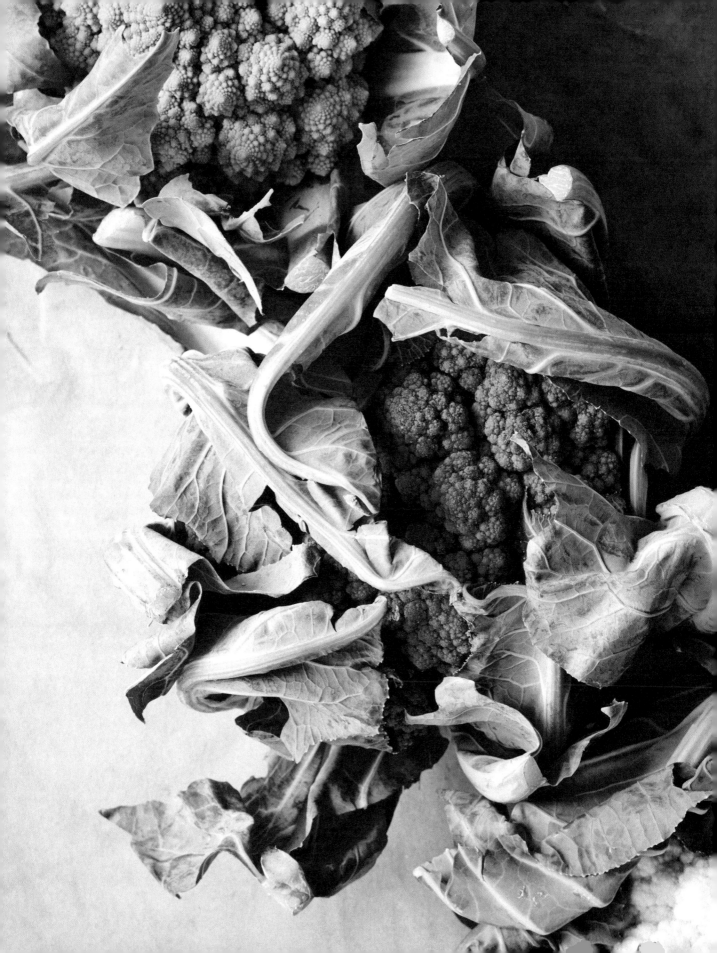

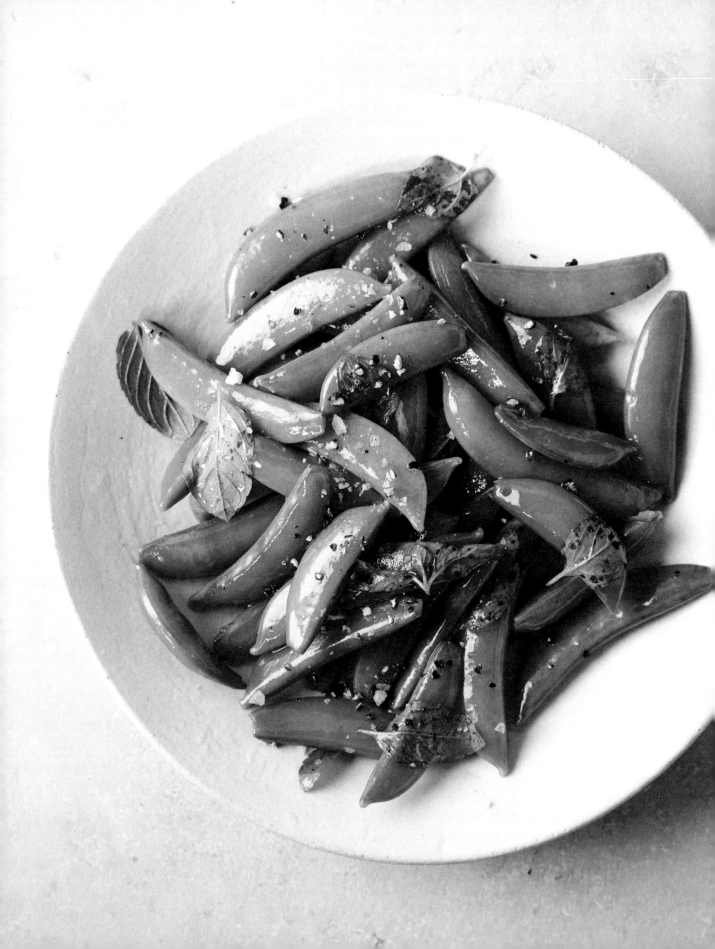

DIANA'S SUGAR SNAP PEAS
with OLIVE OIL and SPEARMINT

SERVES 4, **V, GF**

I promise you that this quick and easy preparation of sugar snap peas will become a summer favorite. Look for pods that are evenly green, firm, and free of blemishes. Observe the usual caution: do not overcook them; better to err on the side of too crunchy than too soft. This is the essence of good, healthy fast food.

1 pound sugar snap peas, stems and strings removed

¼ cup chopped fresh spearmint

2 tablespoons extra-virgin olive oil

½ teaspoon sea salt, or more to taste

Freshly ground black pepper, to taste

1. Place the snap peas in a steamer basket over gently boiling water, cover, and steam for 3 minutes or just until the pods are bright green and crisp-tender. Try a pod a little bit before you think they are done, to avoid overcooking.

2. While the peas are steaming, mix the remaining ingredients in a serving bowl.

3. As soon as the peas are done, turn them into the serving bowl and toss. Taste and adjust with more salt and pepper, if necessary.

QUICK SAUTÉED BEET GREENS

SERVES 4, **V, GF**

This simple preparation of beet greens—quickly sautéed in olive oil, accented with onion, red pepper flakes, and balsamic vinegar—is a nice balance of bitter, sweet, and sour. Note that beet greens are naturally salty. Taste them at the end of cooking to see if they need salt before you add any to the pan.

2 tablespoons extra-virgin olive oil

1 pound beet greens, leaves and stems separated, roughly chopped

1 large onion, thinly sliced

¼ teaspoon crushed red pepper flakes, or more to taste

1 tablespoon balsamic vinegar, or more to taste

1. Heat the oil in a skillet over medium-high heat. Add the beet stems, onion, and red pepper flakes and sauté for 3 to 4 minutes. Add the beet greens and stir-fry just until wilted and tender, another 2 to 3 minutes.

2. Turn off the heat and add the balsamic vinegar. Stir to combine and transfer the greens to a serving dish.

SPICY TOMATO BROCCOLI RABE

SERVES 4, **VEG, V*, GF**

Broccoli rabe, or rapini, is a green cruciferous vegetable, popular in southern Italian cuisine, with edible leaves, stems, and flower buds (the buds resemble broccoli but do not form large heads). All are slightly bitter, a flavor loved in Italy but too often shunned in North America. This easy preparation makes it very tasty.

4 garlic cloves, pressed and allowed to sit for 10 minutes

¼ cup crushed tomatoes

½ cup roasted red peppers (homemade or jarred)

¼ cup finely grated Parmesan cheese, plus more for serving (optional)

⅛ teaspoon crushed red pepper flakes

¼ teaspoon dried oregano

¼ teaspoon grade B maple syrup (optional)

½ teaspoon grated lemon zest

3 tablespoons extra-virgin olive oil

2 teaspoons sea salt

1 pound broccoli rabe

Juice of 1 lemon

1. In a blender or food processor, combine ¾ of the garlic and the next 7 ingredients and process for about 1 minute or until completely smooth. Slowly add 2 tablespoons of the oil and continue blending for another 15 seconds. Transfer this sauce to a jar with tight-fitting lid.

2. Bring a large pot of water to the boil and add the salt. Trim the last 2 inches of fibrous stem off the broccoli rabe, then cut the remaining stems in half lengthwise; this will speed cooking time. Prepare a large ice-water bath.

3. Blanch the broccoli rabe for 1 minute in the boiling water, then immediately transfer it to the prepared ice-water bath. When it is cool, drain it, squeezing out as much water as you can.

4. Heat the remaining 1 tablespoon oil in a skillet over medium heat and add the remaining garlic and 1 tablespoon of the spicy tomato sauce. Add the blanched broccoli rabe to the pan and sauté for 3 minutes.

5. Stir in the remaining spicy tomato sauce and lemon juice and heat briefly. Transfer to a serving dish and garnish with more cheese if you wish.

ZUCCHINI RIBBONS
with BASIL and PARMESAN

SERVES 4, **VEG, GF**

Cutting raw zucchini into thin ribbons and tossing them in a garlic, lemon, and olive oil vinaigrette makes a refreshing summer side dish. A good quantity of shredded fresh basil and the addition of toasted pine nuts are great enhancements.

1½ pounds zucchini, peeled and trimmed

1 cup finely sliced fresh basil leaves

¼ cup toasted pine nuts (page 274)

1 cup Basic Lemon Vinaigrette (page 267)

½ cup shaved or grated Parmesan cheese

1. Working from the top to bottom, peel the zucchini into ribbons using a vegetable peeler or mandolin; the slices should be just about a sixteenth of an inch thick.

2. Place the zucchini, basil, pine nuts, and dressing in a large bowl and gently toss with your hands to evenly coat.

3. Transfer the zucchini to a serving platter, top with the Parmesan, and serve.

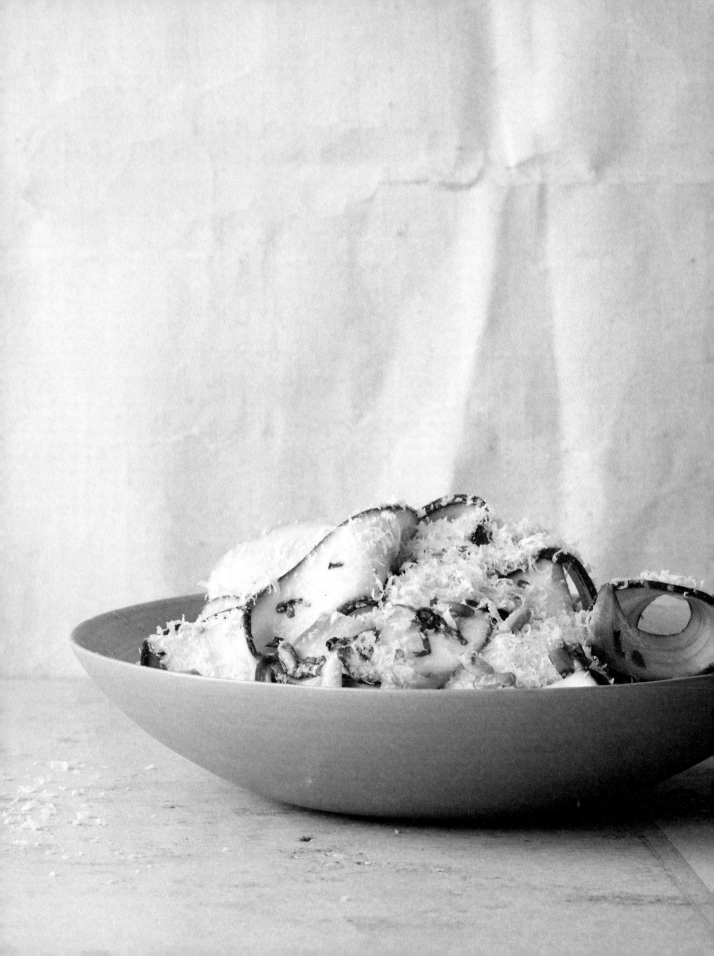

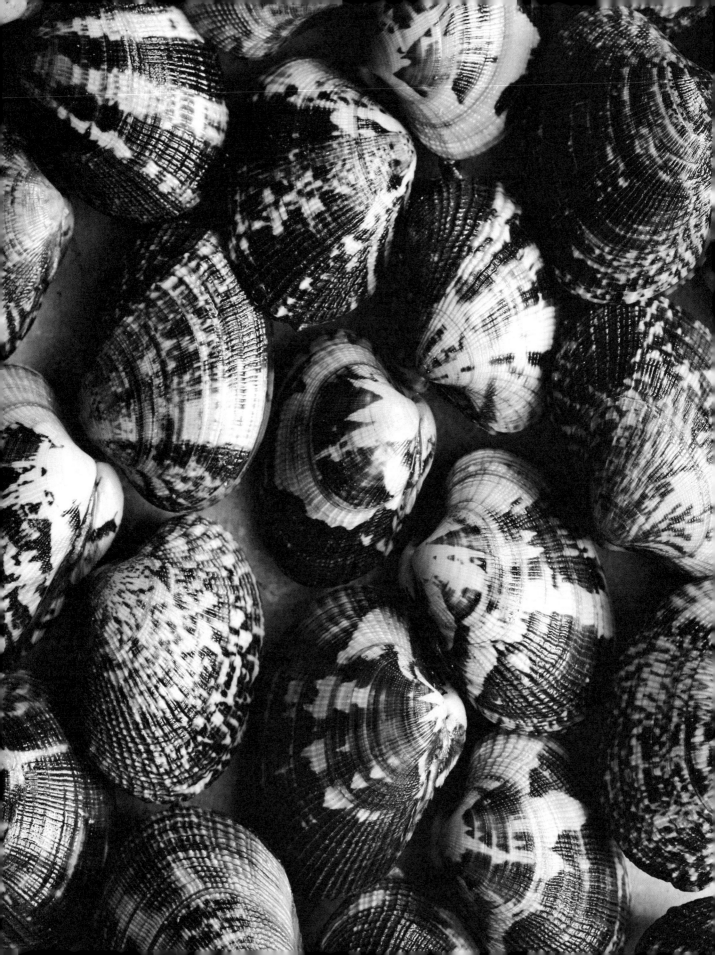

Mains

Now for the main course. Those words create anticipation of the arrival of the meal's centerpiece, the dish that you have spent the most time on and that should live up to expectations. Not long ago, people expected a hunk of animal protein for their main course: a roast, a steak, or fried chicken, for example. You will find a few meat and poultry recipes in this section, but many more feature fish and shellfish, which have a larger place in the Anti-Inflammatory Diet. Other recipes are based on beans and tofu. Consider also recipes in the Pasta and Grains section; many of them make great main courses.

Recipes marked **veg** are vegetarian, those marked **v** are vegan, and those marked **gf** are gluten-free. The symbols **veg***, **v***, and **gf*** indicate recipes that can be modified to be vegetarian, vegan, or gluten-free by substituting or omitting specific ingredients.

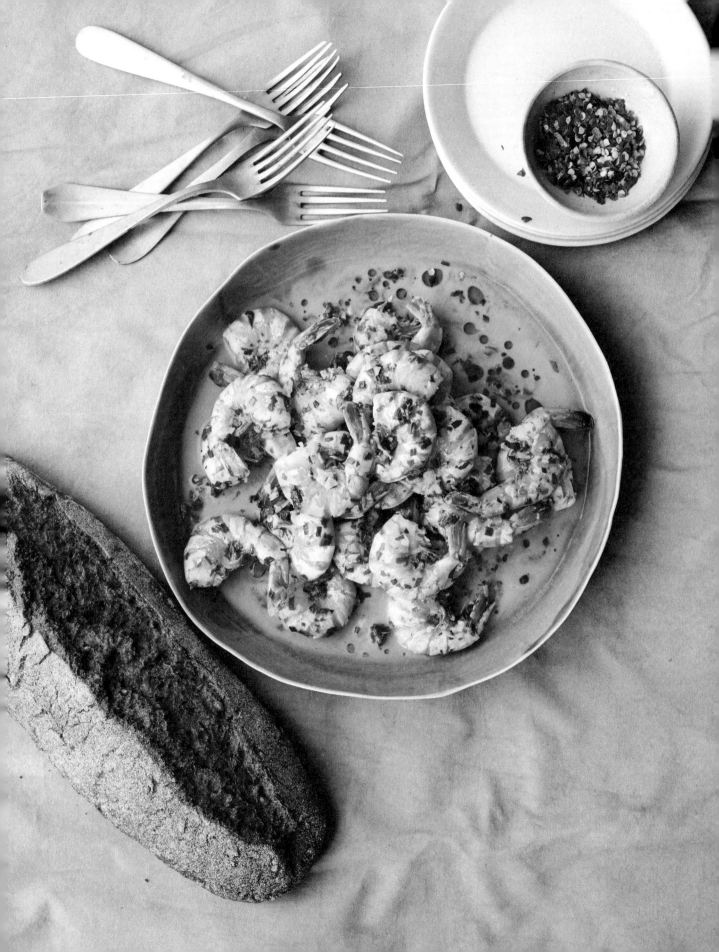

AJAX'S FAVORITE PRAWNS
with GARLIC, HERBS, and WINE

SERVES 4, **GF**

If you're lucky enough to find fresh or frozen wild spot prawns, this is my favorite way to prepare them, but any large wild shrimp will work, as long as you don't overcook them. That's easier to do than you might think, and it greatly diminishes the quality of the dish. The shrimp should be barely cooked through when you turn off the heat, so turn it off slightly before you think they are done. If you have everything ready to go, you and your guests will be in prawn heaven in a matter of minutes. This is messy to eat, but your guests will probably enjoy sucking the meat out of the shells and licking the scrumptious juice from their fingers. (Ajax is my stellar companion animal, a six-year-old Rhodesian ridgeback with refined tastes.)

3 tablespoons extra-virgin olive oil

½ teaspoon crushed red pepper flakes

1 pound shell-on spot prawns or jumbo or large wild shrimp

4 to 5 garlic cloves, pressed and allowed to sit for 10 minutes

½ teaspoon sea salt

2 tablespoons chopped fresh flat-leaf parsley leaves

2 tablespoons chopped fresh basil

2 tablespoons chopped fresh chives

¾ cup dry (white) vermouth

1. Heat the olive oil in a large nonstick skillet over medium-high heat. When hot, add the red pepper flakes, prawns, and garlic. Sauté the prawns until they begin to turn pink and curl, about 2 minutes. Sprinkle with salt, add the herbs and vermouth, and let the prawns cook for 1 more minute, until they are just cooked through and the liquid is somewhat reduced. Remove from the heat.

2. Divide the shrimp and any sauce among 4 bowls. Serve immediately, with an extra bowl to discard the prawn shells and, if you wish, good crusty bread to sop up the flavorful liquid.

GRILLED MAHI-MAHI with CHERMOULA

SERVES 4, GF

Chermoula is a marinade or sauce made of herbs, spices, and citrus that is used with seafood in Algerian, Tunisian, and Moroccan cooking. It is easy to make and bursting with flavor. Here it turns simple grilled fish into a memorable main course.

CHERMOULA

4 garlic cloves, pressed and allowed to sit for 10 minutes

1 teaspoon sea salt

2 bunches fresh flat-leaf parsley, leaves picked (about 2 cups)

3 bunches fresh cilantro, leaves picked (about 3 cups)

1 tablespoon cumin seeds, toasted and ground

¾ teaspoon coriander seeds, toasted and ground

1½ teaspoons sweet paprika

¼ teaspoon cayenne pepper

½ cup extra-virgin olive oil

¼ cup lemon juice

FISH

4 (6-ounce) skinless mahi-mahi fillets at room temperature

Sea salt

Freshly ground black pepper

4 teaspoons grapeseed oil

Lemon wedges

1. Place all the chermoula ingredients in a blender and blend until the mixture reaches a coarse puree.

2. Pat the fish fillets dry and season them on both sides with salt and black pepper. Place the fillets in a large baking dish with ½ cup of the chermoula. Rub the sauce into the fish with your hands, cover, and refrigerate for at least 15 minutes.

3. Preheat a grill pan or grill over medium heat. Rub each piece of fish with 1 teaspoon of grapeseed oil. Place the fish on the grill and cook for 5 minutes, or until the fish does not stick to the grill. (You should be able to easily lift the corner of the fish before you flip it over.) Flip the fish and cook for 3 more minutes or until firm to the touch. Remove from the grill and transfer to plates.

4. Serve the fish with the remaining chermoula sauce on the side, along with a lemon wedge.

CIOPPINO

SERVES 8, **GF***

Cioppino is a tomato-based Italian-American seafood stew that originated in San Francisco. Many versions exist but all are mixtures of finfish and shellfish in a rich tomato broth flavored with wine, garlic, and red pepper. Be careful not to overcook the seafood, and serve the cioppino immediately. It is messy to eat, so provide plenty of paper towels and bowls for discarded shells. Although restaurants always serve this with lots of bread, that's not necessary. Even without bread, cioppino is a filling one-dish meal.

3 tablespoons extra-virgin olive oil

2 onions, finely chopped

1 large carrot, peeled and finely grated

½ teaspoon plus a pinch of sea salt

6 garlic cloves, pressed and allowed to sit for 10 minutes, plus 4 cloves, halved (optional)

¼ teaspoon crushed red pepper flakes

2 tablespoons tomato paste

12 ounces clam juice

1 cup dry white wine

4 to 5 cups seafood stock, Quick Vegetable Stock (page 266), or store-bought vegetable broth

½ cup fresh flat-leaf parsley leaves, finely chopped

12 littleneck clams, scrubbed

8 ounces mussels, scrubbed

8 ounces sea scallops, quartered

8 ounces halibut or Pacific cod fillet, cut into 1-inch cubes

12 ounces large shell-on shrimp, deveined

1 cup finely sliced fresh basil leaves

8 slices whole-wheat sourdough bread (optional)

1. Heat the oil in a large pot over medium-high heat, add the onions and carrot with a pinch of salt, and sauté until the onions soften, about 4 minutes. Add the pressed garlic and red pepper flakes and cook for a minute more. Add the tomato paste and stir to combine. Add the clam juice, white wine, 2 cups of the stock, half the parsley, and ½ teaspoon of the salt. Stir to combine and bring to a low boil. Continue to cook over medium heat, uncovered, for 6 to 8 minutes or until the mixture reduces by about half.

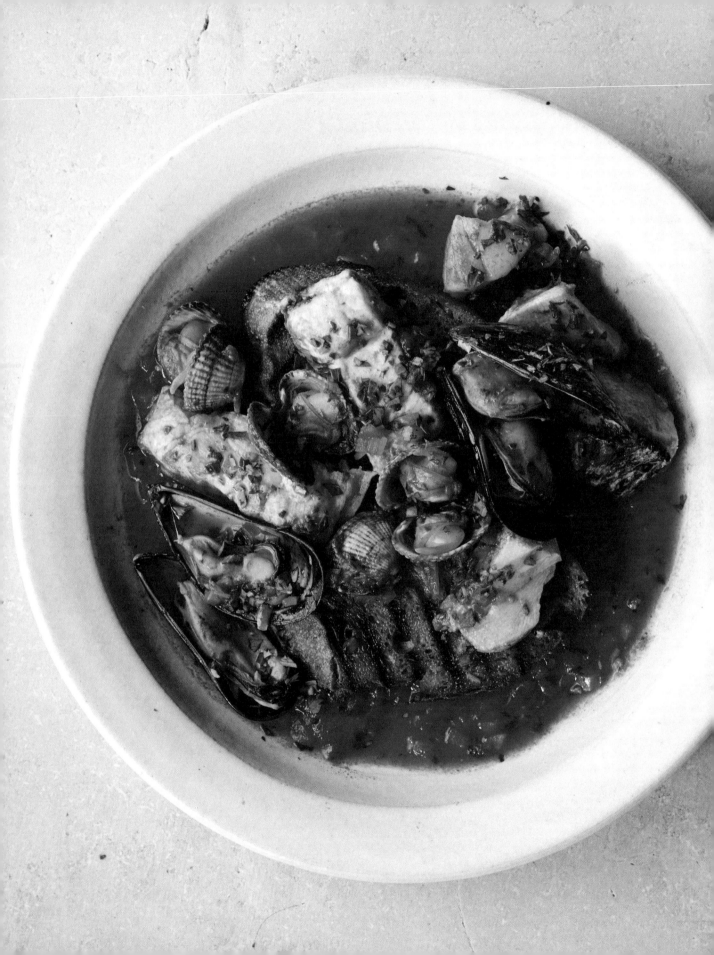

2. Add the clams, cover the pot, and cook for 5 to 6 minutes. Remove the lid and add 1 more cup of the stock and the mussels, scallops, and halibut. Gently toss the seafood with a wooden spoon and cover the pot. Cook just until the clams begin to open. Stir in the shrimp and cook until they are pink and opaque, about 1 to 2 minutes.

3. Turn off the heat and fold in the sliced basil. If the cioppino base is too thick, add more hot broth until the desired consistency is reached.

4. Toast the bread and rub each piece with half a clove of raw garlic.

5. Ladle the cioppino into 8 bowls and sprinkle the remaining parsley over the seafood. Serve hot with the garlic toast.

GRILLED HALIBUT TACOS
with AVOCADO CHIPOTLE CREMA

SERVES 6

Fish tacos, a staple of beach cafés and food carts in Mexico, have become immensely popular here, appearing on the menus of both fast-casual and upscale restaurants. They can be terrific or terrible, mostly depending on the quality and preparation of the fish and the freshness and flavor of the accompanying ingredients. I like fish tacos made with simply grilled firm white fish, chopped raw veggies, and a couple of zingy sauces all wrapped in warm corn tortillas.

2 pounds skinless halibut fillets (about ¾ inch thick)

3 tablespoons grapeseed oil

7 tablespoons lime juice

4 tablespoons adobo sauce (from a can of chipotle peppers in adobo)

3 garlic cloves, pressed and allowed to sit for 10 minutes

2 teaspoons chili powder

1 teaspoon ground cumin

Sea salt and freshly ground black pepper, to taste

2 avocados

2 jalapeño peppers, seeded and finely chopped

1 large white onion, finely diced

2 tomatoes, seeded and diced

1 bunch fresh cilantro, leaves picked and roughly chopped

12 corn tortillas

½ head green cabbage, finely shredded

Hot sauce, to taste

Lime wedges

1. Heat a grill pan or grill over medium heat. Preheat the oven to 350°F.

2. Rub the fish fillets with the grapeseed oil, 2 tablespoons of the lime juice, 2 tablespoons of the adobo sauce, and the garlic and season on all sides with chili powder, cumin, salt, and pepper. Allow the fish to sit at room temperature for at least 5 minutes before cooking.

3. To make the avocado *crema*, mash the avocado, remaining 2 tablespoons adobo sauce, and 2 tablespoons of the lime juice until smooth. Season with salt and set aside.

4. To make the fresh salsa, mix the jalapeños, onions, tomatoes, half of the cilantro, and the remaining lime juice together and set aside.

5. Grill the fish for 5 to 6 minutes, without turning, until brown. While the fish cooks, wrap the tortillas in foil and warm them in the oven. Carefully flip the fillets and cook for 2 to 3 minutes more or until just cooked through and opaque. Transfer the fish to a serving dish, let it rest for a moment, and then cut the fillets into 3- to 4-inch pieces.

6. To assemble a taco, place a piece of fish in a warm tortilla and top with some cabbage, fresh salsa, avocado *crema*, and cilantro. Serve with hot sauce and a lime wedge.

GINGER-SCALLION STEAMED SEA BASS

SERVES 4, GF

Steaming is an ideal and much underused way to cook. It is the most energy-efficient method and the one least likely to create the toxic compounds formed when foods, especially animal protein, are cooked at high temperatures. Steaming is particularly appropriate for fish, because it reduces the chance of overcooking and keeps it moist. Here, a mild-fleshed fish is quickly steamed with typical Asian flavors.

2 garlic cloves, pressed and allowed to sit for 10 minutes

¼ cup Shaoxing wine or dry sherry

1 (3-inch) piece fresh ginger, peels reserved, ginger cut into thin shreds

4 (5-ounce) sea bass or red snapper fillets

Sea salt and freshly ground pepper, to taste

5 large scallions, cut into 3-inch pieces, then cut lengthwise into strips

2 limes, thinly sliced

¼ cup low-sodium soy sauce

1 tablespoon toasted sesame oil

1. In a shallow pot or wok that fits your steamer basket, combine the garlic, ½ cup of water, wine, and ginger peels. The basket should sit an inch or two above the liquid. Cover the pot and bring to a simmer.

2. With a paper towel, pat the fillets dry and sprinkle with salt and pepper. Cut a circle of parchment paper that will cover the bottom of the steamer basket and cut a 1-inch hole in the center.

3. Place the parchment at the bottom of the basket and evenly lay down half of the scallions, half of the ginger, and half the lime slices. Lay the fish fillets on top of that (it's fine if they overlap), then drizzle with the soy sauce and sesame oil. Top with the remaining scallions, ginger, and lime slices.

4. Place the basket in the pot, cover, and steam for about 5 to 6 minutes or until the fish are opaque in the center. Remove the covered basket and set aside. Turn up the heat and reduce the liquid slightly, about 2 minutes. Add more water, a tablespoon at a time, if the liquid is reducing too quickly.

5. Carefully move the fish to 4 plates and drizzle a few spoonfuls of the reduction over each piece. Garnish with the steamed scallions and ginger and serve with Forbidden Rice with Ginger and Lemongrass (page 195) or your favorite rice or grain.

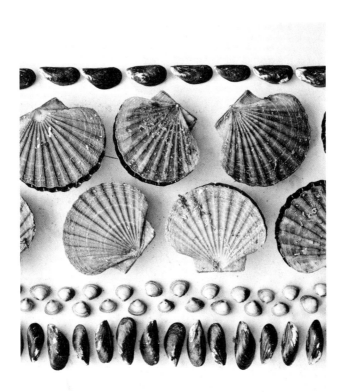

FISH COOKED in PARCHMENT
with ORANGE, SESAME, and GINGER

SERVES 4, **GF**

Baking in parchment is a foolproof and healthful way to cook fish, leaving it moist and always delicious. Even the most delicate fish never seems to be dry when prepared this way, and it comes to the table with style. If you're having company, prepare the packets an hour or two in advance, then preheat the oven when you're ready. This recipe can also be scaled down to a single serving faster than you can say *takeout*.

¼ cup low-sodium soy sauce

2 tablespoons freshly squeezed orange juice

1 tablespoon unseasoned rice vinegar

2 teaspoons fish sauce

2 teaspoons toasted sesame oil

1 tablespoon minced or grated peeled ginger

8 shiitake mushrooms, stemmed and thinly sliced

4 (6-ounce) skinless white fish fillets (sea bass, cod, or halibut)

1 teaspoon sea salt

½ teaspoon freshly ground black pepper

2 oranges, thinly sliced (12 slices)

2 tablespoons finely chopped fresh cilantro

4 scallions, white and light green parts only, thinly sliced on the bias

1. Preheat the oven to 400°F.

2. In a small bowl, combine the soy sauce, orange juice, rice vinegar, fish sauce, and sesame oil. Stir in the minced ginger and sliced mushrooms and set aside.

3. Season both sides of the fish with salt and pepper.

4. Tear off an 18-inch sheet of parchment paper and fold it in half. Draw half a large heart on the paper. Cut the paper so you have a full heart when the paper is unfolded. On the left side of the heart, place 3 of the orange slices, then put one fish fillet on top. Spoon ¼ of the sauce on top of the fish. Fold the other half of the parchment heart over the fish. Seal the package by making overlapping folds, one on top of the other, about 10 folds, until the opposite corner of the folded edge is reached. Twist the last fold at the end of the paper several times to make a tight seal and tuck it under the packet. Repeat for the remaining fish fillets.

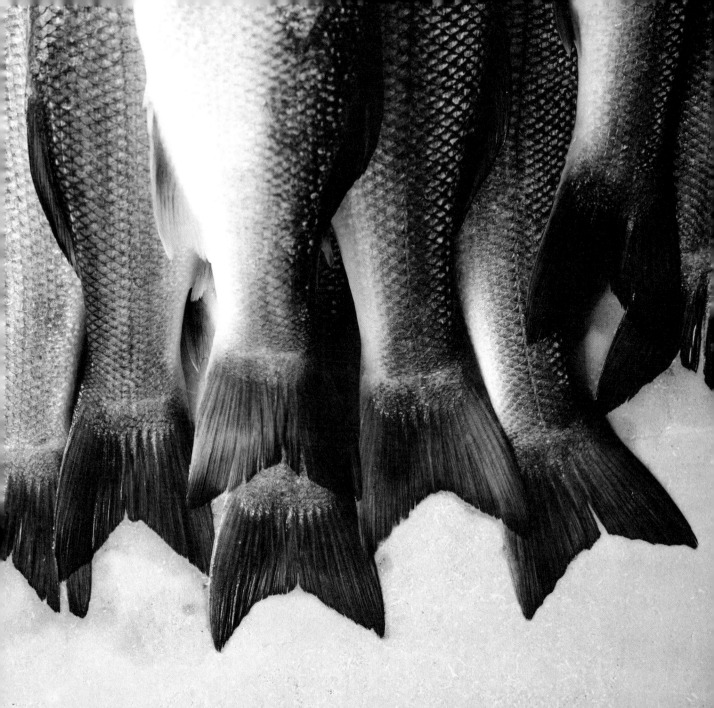

5. Place the packets on a baking sheet and bake until the paper turns brown around the edge and puffs up, about 10 to 12 minutes.

6. Transfer each package to a plate. Carefully cut an X in the top of each to allow the steam to escape. For the full visual effect, cut each package open at the table. Top each serving with cilantro and scallions.

BISTRO-STYLE MUSSELS

SERVES 4

Mussels have many things going for them: they are inexpensive, quick to cook, and a good source of both omega-3 fatty acids and vitamin B12. This is a classic preparation with a twist: extra-virgin olive oil takes the place of the butter that French recipes call for. Buy mussels from a dealer who can assure you of their freshness, get them home quickly, put them in a bowl, place a damp towel on them to keep them from drying out, and put them in the refrigerator. Cook them as soon as possible—certainly within a day of purchase. Scrub them well with a stiff brush to clean them.

2 tablespoons extra-virgin olive oil

2 shallots, finely chopped

Pinch of sea salt

Freshly ground black pepper

2 garlic cloves, pressed and allowed to sit for 10 minutes

1 Turkish bay leaf or ⅓ of a California bay leaf

1 teaspoon dried whole thyme leaves

1 cup dry (white) vermouth or dry white wine

2 pounds mussels, scrubbed

3 tablespoons chopped fresh flat-leaf parsley leaves

Crusty whole-grain bread

1. In a large pot, heat the olive oil over medium-high heat. Add the shallots, a pinch of salt, and a few grinds of black pepper and sauté for 1 minute. Add the garlic and continue sautéing for another minute. Add the bay leaf, thyme, and wine and bring to a boil. Add the mussels, cover the pot, and cook for about 3 to 4 minutes or until most of the mussels open. (Discard any that have not opened.)

2. Transfer the mussels and cooking liquid to a large bowl and scatter the chopped parsley over them. Serve with crusty bread to soak up the flavorful liquid.

NIGELLA'S EASIEST MIRIN SALMON

SERVES 4, **GF**

Nigella Lawson's recipe for mirin-glazed salmon became an instant classic. It's a foolproof way to prepare salmon fillets so that they turn out perfectly cooked and totally delicious. I'm indebted to her for it. To make it consistent with the nutritional philosophy of this book, I've cut the amount of sugar she calls for.

¼ cup mirin

2 tablespoons evaporated cane sugar

¼ cup low-sodium soy sauce

4 (4-ounce) skinless salmon fillets, about 1 inch thick

2 tablespoons unseasoned rice vinegar

1 to 2 scallions, white and light green parts only, thinly sliced lengthwise

1. Whisk the mirin, sugar, and soy sauce together in a bowl until the sugar is dissolved. Place the salmon in a shallow dish and pour the marinade over the fish. Marinate for 3 minutes, then turn over and marinate the other side for an additional 2 minutes.

2. Heat a nonstick pan over medium-high heat. When hot, remove the fish from the marinade (reserve the marinade) and place it presentation-side down in the pan. Cook, undisturbed, for 2 minutes. Turn the salmon over, pour the reserved marinade over it, and cook for another 2 minutes.

3. Remove the fillets to serving plates. Add the rice vinegar to the mixture in the pan and cook to reduce it by about half. Pour the dark, sweet, salty glaze over the salmon and top with the scallion strips. Serve with rice or noodles as you wish, and consider putting some pickled ginger on the table too (available from Japanese food stores and online).

BROILED HALIBUT with GREEN HARISSA

SERVES 4, GF

Halibut is a delicate fish that's easy to cook under the broiler, a method that seals its surface and renders the interior moist and flaky. It's also a blank canvas for a great sauce, such as this green harissa, which combines Middle Eastern spices with a little south-of-the-border jalapeño. I find that even people who think they don't like fish love this dish.

GREEN HARISSA

1 garlic clove, pressed and allowed to sit for 10 minutes

½ cup fresh cilantro leaves

¼ cup fresh flat-leaf parsley leaves

¼ cup extra-virgin olive oil

¼ cup lemon juice

½ teaspoon ground cumin

¼ teaspoon ground coriander

1 jalapeño pepper, seeded and sliced

¼ teaspoon sea salt

HALIBUT

4 (6-ounce) halibut fillets

½ teaspoon sea salt

1 tablespoon grapeseed oil

1. Put all the harissa ingredients in a food processor and process until smooth. Transfer to a small bowl and reserve.

2. Preheat the broiler to high.

3. Pat the halibut fillets dry with a paper towel and season both sides with salt. Place an ovenproof skillet large enough to hold the fish in a single layer on the stove over medium-high heat. When the pan is hot, heat the grapeseed oil. Lay the fish in the hot pan and immediately place it under the broiler. Cook until golden brown or to the desired doneness, 8 to 10 minutes. Transfer the fish onto 4 plates and top each piece with 2 tablespoons of the harissa. Store any unused harissa in an airtight jar in the refrigerator for up to a week.

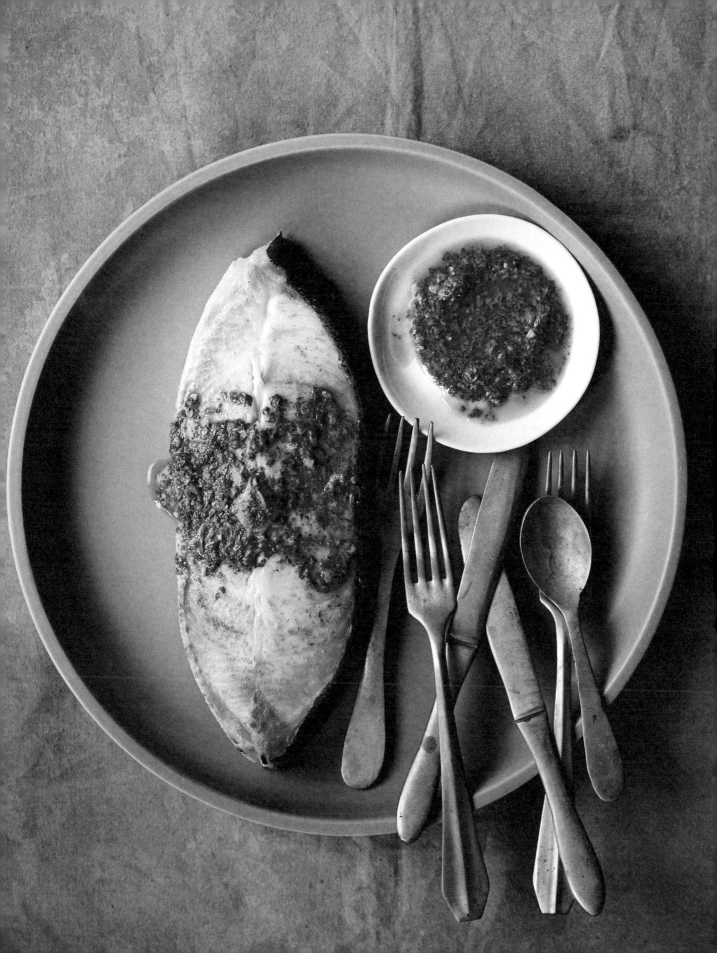

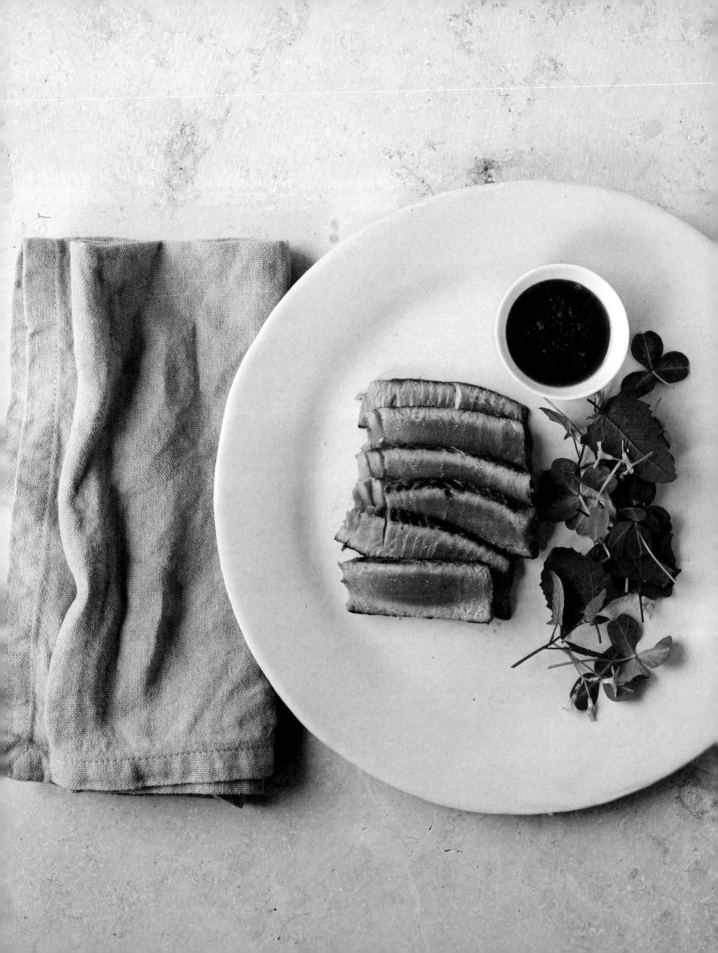

PAN-SEARED ALBACORE TUNA LOIN

SERVES 4, **GF**

I think albacore tuna loin is best cooked rare with a thin seared outer layer, but loins are usually thicker in the middle with tapered ends, so there will be more-done and less-done portions that will suit individual preferences. The marinade gives a classic Japanese flavor to the fish. If you're in a hurry, even 30 minutes of marinating will do the job. Tuna cooked this way doesn't need any condiment, but if you wish, you can serve it with wasabi paste and pickled ginger (both available from Japanese food stores and online).

MARINADE

3 garlic cloves, pressed and allowed to sit for 10 minutes

1 cup sake

⅔ cup low-sodium soy sauce

2 tablespoons evaporated cane sugar

1-inch piece ginger root, peeled and grated

1 tablespoon toasted sesame oil

TUNA LOIN

4 (6-ounce) pieces albacore tuna loin (thawed completely if frozen)

3 tablespoons grapeseed oil

1. Mix the marinade ingredients until the sugar dissolves. Pour half the marinade over the tuna in a shallow dish, then cover. Place the tuna in the refrigerator for at least 30 minutes, turning occasionally to make sure all of it is flavored with the marinade.

2. Remove the tuna from the refrigerator 20 minutes before cooking.

3. In a small saucepan, bring the remaining marinade and 2 tablespoons of water to a gentle boil and allow it to reduce a little. Reserve.

4. Heat the grapeseed oil in a nonstick skillet over high heat until hot but not smoking.

5. Place the tuna in the hot oil and sear on each side to desired doneness. For rare, this may be just 2 minutes on each side. (Check the ends or slice through the middle to check doneness.)

6. Remove the tuna loin to a heated platter and cut into ½- to 1-inch slices, as desired. Drizzle the sauce over the tuna and serve immediately.

ROASTED SALMON TOPPED
with SAKE-GLAZED SHIITAKE

SERVES 4, **GF**

Fresh salmon fillets are baked gently and smothered with a flavorful preparation of shiitake mushrooms. Quick and simple but also elegant, this is a main course for any occasion. The salmon must not be dry; be careful not to overcook it.

4 (6-ounce) salmon fillets, pinbones removed

Spritz of lime juice, plus more for finishing

½ teaspoon sea salt

¼ teaspoon freshly ground black pepper

2 tablespoons grapeseed oil

4 ounces shiitake mushrooms, stemmed and sliced

2 garlic cloves, pressed and allowed to sit for 10 minutes

1 tablespoon minced peeled fresh ginger

⅓ cup seeded and diced red bell pepper

⅓ cup sake

2 scallions, white and light green parts only, chopped

1. Preheat the oven to 325°F and line a rimmed baking sheet with parchment paper.

2. Place the fish on the baking sheet and sprinkle with the lime juice, half the salt, and half the pepper. Roast for 12 to 13 minutes or until just opaque. Don't be afraid to take the fish out a little before you think it's done since it will continue to cook once you remove it from the oven.

3. While the fish bakes, heat the oil in a 10- or 12-inch skillet over medium-high heat. Add the shiitake and the remaining salt and pepper and cook until softened and slightly browned, about 5 minutes. Add the garlic and ginger, stirring until just fragrant, about 20 seconds. Stir in the red pepper and sake and reduce the liquid for about 1 minute or until the sake begins to bubble up around the edge of the pan. Remove from the heat.

4. To serve, top each piece of salmon with mushrooms, a squeeze of lime juice, and some of the scallions.

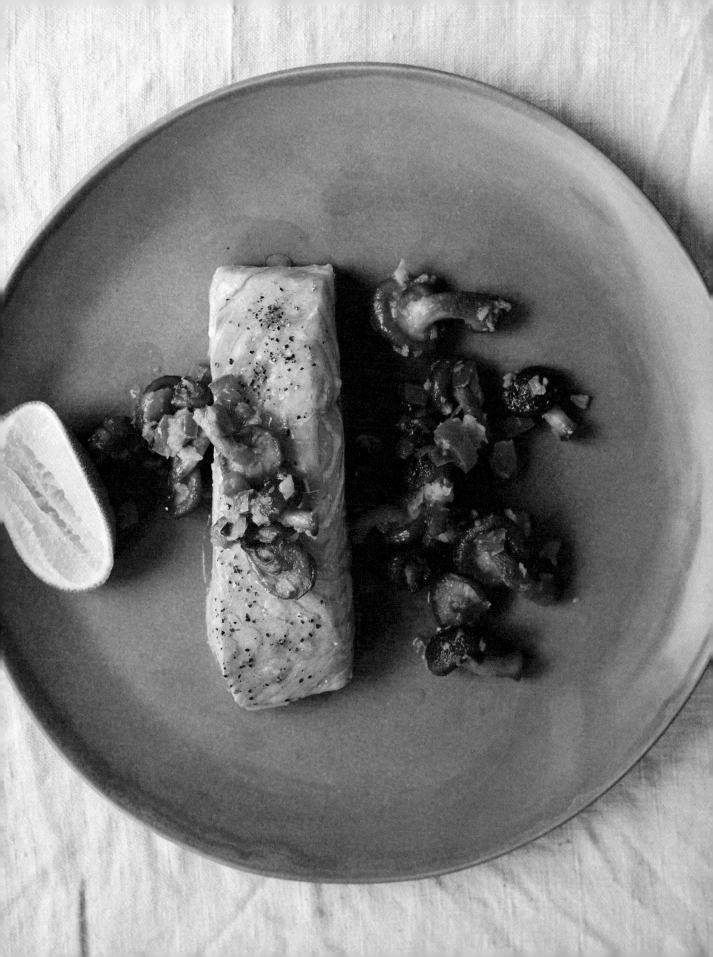

PAN-SEARED SCALLOPS
with STIR-FRIED BABY BOK CHOY

SERVES 4, GF

Perfect pan-seared scallops should be caramelized on the surface and just cooked through so that they are tender and sweet. This very simple method does the job right every time. A bed of stir-fried bok choy and mushrooms makes for a beautiful presentation.

3 tablespoons grapeseed oil

4 garlic cloves, pressed and allowed to sit for 10 minutes

2 teaspoons grated peeled ginger

6 ounces shiitake mushrooms, stemmed and sliced

1 pound baby bok choy, leaves and stems separated

1½ tablespoons low-sodium soy sauce, or to taste

1 teaspoon toasted sesame oil

1¼ pounds large diver scallops

Sea salt and freshly ground black pepper, to taste

Juice of half a lemon

1. Heat 2 tablespoons of the grapeseed oil in a large skillet over medium-high heat. Add the garlic and ginger and stir-fry for 30 seconds. Add the mushrooms and cook for 2 minutes, being careful not to burn the garlic. Add the bok choy and sauté for 3 to 4 minutes.

2. Turn off the heat and stir in the soy sauce and toasted sesame oil. Transfer the bok choy to a platter and keep warm.

3. Wipe out the pan and add the remaining 1 tablespoon grapeseed oil. Place over medium-high heat. Pat the scallops dry with a paper towel and sprinkle salt and pepper on one side. When the oil is hot (but not smoking), place the scallops in the pan, seasoned-side down.

4. Do not touch the scallops as they cook. Cook for 3 minutes if scallops are less than an inch thick, 4 minutes if thicker. Sprinkle salt and pepper on the unseasoned sides and turn the scallops over. Cook for the same amount of time on the second side, undisturbed, until nicely browned.

5. Turn off the heat and squeeze the lemon juice over the scallops. Transfer the scallops immediately to the bed of bok choy and serve.

PERSIAN TURKEY SLIDERS
with YOGURT-TAHINI SAUCE

SERVES 8, GF*

The Middle Eastern spice mixture transforms what could be a bland turkey experience into something really tasty, and the yogurt-tahini sauce takes it over the top. The key to a tender burger—one that doesn't resemble a hockey puck—is using a light hand when combining the turkey with the other ingredients.

SLIDERS

3 garlic cloves, pressed and allowed to sit for 10 minutes

½ cup finely chopped onion

2 tablespoons coarsely chopped fresh flat-leaf parsley leaves

1 teaspoon ground cumin

½ teaspoon ground coriander

½ teaspoon sea salt

¼ teaspoon ground cinnamon

⅛ teaspoon cayenne pepper

1 pound ground dark turkey meat

1 tablespoon grapeseed oil

8 lettuce leaves

8 slices tomato

4 whole-wheat pita pockets, halved (optional)

YOGURT-TAHINI SAUCE

¼ cup plain Greek yogurt

2 tablespoons tahini

1 teaspoon grated lemon zest

1 to 2 tablespoons lemon juice

⅛ teaspoon sea salt

Pinch of cayenne pepper

¼ cup peeled, seeded, and finely chopped cucumber

1 tablespoon finely chopped fresh spearmint

1. Put the garlic, onion, parsley, cumin, coriander, salt, cinnamon, and cayenne in a large bowl and stir to combine. Add the turkey and gently mix with your hands or a spatula until well combined. Shape the mixture into 8 patties (each about the size of your palm).

2. To make the sauce, whisk together the yogurt, tahini, lemon zest, lemon juice, salt, and cayenne in a bowl. Stir in 1 to 2 teaspoons of water, as needed, to achieve a spoonable consistency. Fold in the cucumber and spearmint.

3. Preheat a grill pan over medium heat. Brush with the grapeseed oil, then put the patties in the pan and cook until browned on both sides, about 3 minutes per side. Add 1 tablespoon of water, cover, and cook for 3 more minutes, or until an instant-read thermometer registers 165°F. Alternatively, heat a skillet over medium heat, add just enough oil to coat the skillet, then put the patties in the skillet and cook until browned on both sides, about 3 minutes on each side. Decrease the heat to medium-low, add 1 tablespoon of water, cover, and cook for 3 minutes more.

4. Transfer the sliders to plates and serve with a generous dollop of yogurt-tahini sauce, lettuce leaves, tomatoes, and warmed pita, if desired.

SOUTHWESTERN TURKEY CHILI

SERVES 4, V*, GF

Commercial chili powder is a mixture of dried spices: oregano, garlic, ground cumin, and red chili, usually with added salt. These are the basic flavor elements of the many varieties of the popular stew called chili that may or may not contain beans. I often make a vegan chili from dried, soaked adzuki beans, which cook quickly, sometimes adding sautéed shiitake mushrooms for their meaty texture. You can serve this as a one-dish meal, letting guests add chopped tomatoes, onions, and shredded cheese as they wish. Warm corn tortillas are also a good accompaniment.

1 tablespoon extra-virgin olive oil

1 large yellow onion, diced

½ teaspoon sea salt

2 garlic cloves, pressed and allowed to sit for 10 minutes

1 jalapeño pepper, seeded and minced

1 red bell pepper, seeded and diced

1 teaspoon dried oregano

2 teaspoons ground cumin

2 teaspoons smoked paprika

⅛ teaspoon cayenne pepper, or more to taste

¼ teaspoon ground allspice

½ pound lean ground turkey or crumbled tempeh

1 (14.5-ounce) can diced tomatoes with their juice

1 (15-ounce) can black beans, rinsed and drained

¼ teaspoon lime juice

2 tablespoons chopped fresh cilantro leaves

1. In a soup pot, heat the oil over medium heat. Add the onions and a pinch of salt and sauté for 3 minutes, until translucent. Add the garlic, jalapeño, red pepper, oregano, and spices and sauté for another minute.

2. Add the turkey and ¼ teaspoon of the salt. Break up the meat with a wooden spoon and let it brown, about 3 minutes. If pan is dry or the spices stick, pour in a little juice from the tomatoes to deglaze.

3. Add the tomatoes, beans, and another pinch of salt. Stir to combine. Bring the chili to a simmer, then lower heat, cover, and simmer for 20 minutes, stirring occasionally. Remove the lid and simmer for 10 minutes more, stirring occasionally. Add the lime juice and a generous pinch of salt, to taste.

4. Ladle the chili into 4 bowls and garnish with cilantro and your favorite accompaniments.

ANDY'S ANYTIME TOFU SCRAMBLE
with SALSA CRUDA

SERVES 4, **V, GF***

This is a good breakfast dish and can also be a clean-out-the-refrigerator meal, since you can add any vegetables you have on hand. Turmeric gives an appealing color and cumin a rich flavor. It's fun to scoop the scramble up in warm, soft corn tortillas, but feel free to omit them and just dig in.

2 tablespoons grapeseed oil

1 small onion, diced

3 tablespoons diced red bell pepper

3 garlic cloves, pressed and allowed to sit for 10 minutes

16 ounces extra-firm tofu, drained and crumbled into small pieces

1 teaspoon turmeric

½ teaspoon ground cumin

1 teaspoon sea salt

⅛ teaspoon cayenne pepper

4 corn tortillas (optional)

1 avocado, thinly sliced (optional)

Fresh Salsa Cruda (page 170) (optional)

1. Preheat the oven to 350°F.

2. In a large skillet, heat the oil over medium-high heat. Add the onion and diced pepper and sauté until the onion is translucent, about 2 minutes. Stir in the garlic, and sauté for 30 seconds more. Add the tofu, then add the turmeric, cumin, salt, and cayenne and cook for 3 more minutes, stirring occasionally.

3. Place the tortillas on a cookie sheet and bake for 5 minutes until warmed through. (Or wrap the tortillas in a tea towel and heat them in the microwave for 45 seconds.)

4. Serve the scramble with the warm tortillas, sliced avocados, and salsa.

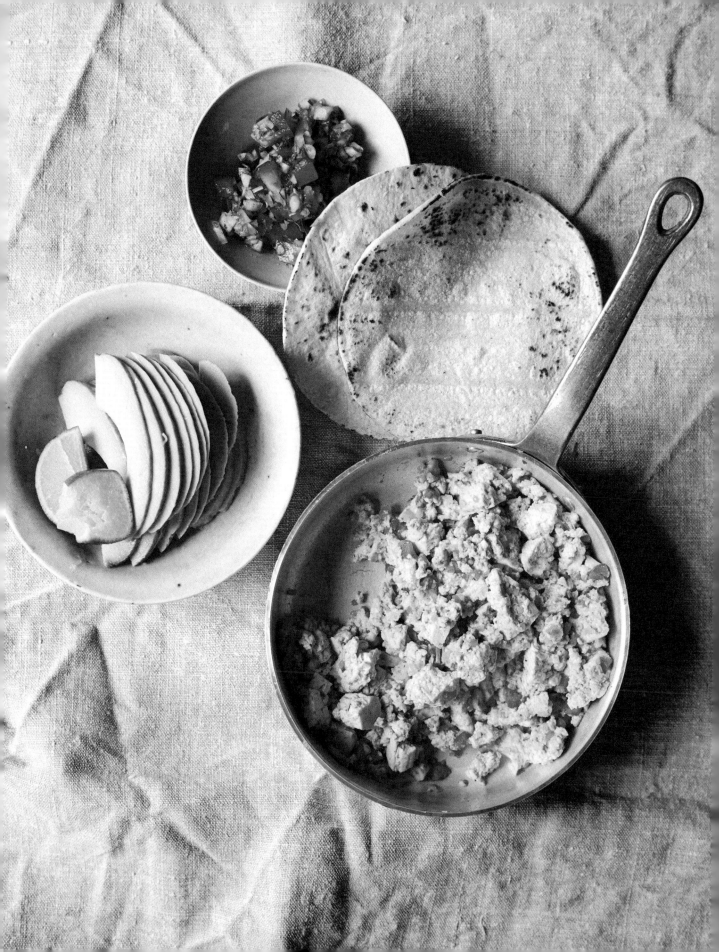

FRESH SALSA CRUDA
MAKES 2 CUPS

½ cup tightly packed cilantro leaves, coarsely chopped

1 cup chopped tomatoes

¼ cup diced red bell pepper

¼ cup diced red onion

1 small jalapeño pepper, seeded and minced

2 tablespoons lime juice

Mix all the ingredients in a medium bowl until thoroughly blended. Cover and refrigerate until ready to use; may be kept for up to 3 days.

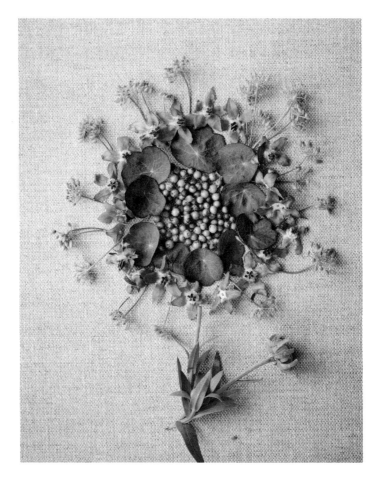

SPICY SICHUAN CHICKEN (or TOFU) STIR-FRY

SERVES 4, **V***, **GF**

This spicy stir-fry, inspired by the cuisine of Sichuan Province in southwestern China, can be made with chicken or baked pressed tofu. It gets its heat from Sriracha sauce.

CHICKEN

4 boneless, skinless chicken thighs, cut into ½-inch pieces, or ½ pound baked pressed tofu, sliced into ½-inch pieces

2 garlic cloves, pressed and allowed to sit for 10 minutes

1 tablespoon minced peeled ginger

½ teaspoon sea salt

¼ teaspoon toasted sesame oil

2 tablespoons grapeseed oil

½ yellow onion, thinly sliced

2 carrots, peeled and thinly sliced on the bias

2 celery stalks, thinly sliced on the bias

1 red bell pepper, seeded and cut into ½-inch cubes

1½ cups (about 4 ounces) snow peas, strings removed

½ cup toasted cashews (page 274)

¼ cup roughly chopped fresh cilantro leaves

2 scallions, white and green parts only, thinly sliced

SPICY STIR-FRY SAUCE

2 tablespoons Sriracha sauce

2 tablespoons lime juice

1½ tablespoons low-sodium soy sauce

1 tablespoon grade B maple syrup

2 teaspoons unseasoned rice vinegar

1 teaspoon toasted sesame oil

1. In a medium bowl, combine the chicken with the garlic, ginger, salt, and sesame oil and allow it to marinate for 15 minutes while you're preparing the rest of the dish.

2. Whisk together the sauce ingredients and set aside.

3. Heat the grapeseed oil in a large wide pan over high heat. Add the chicken and stir-fry for 3 minutes. Add the onions, carrots, and celery and sauté for 2 minutes. Add the peppers and snow peas and stir-fry for 2 minutes more. Add the sauce to the pan and stir to coat. Cook until the sauce begins to reduce a bit, about 1 minute.

4. Transfer the stir-fry onto a platter. Garnish with cashews, cilantro, and scallions and serve hot.

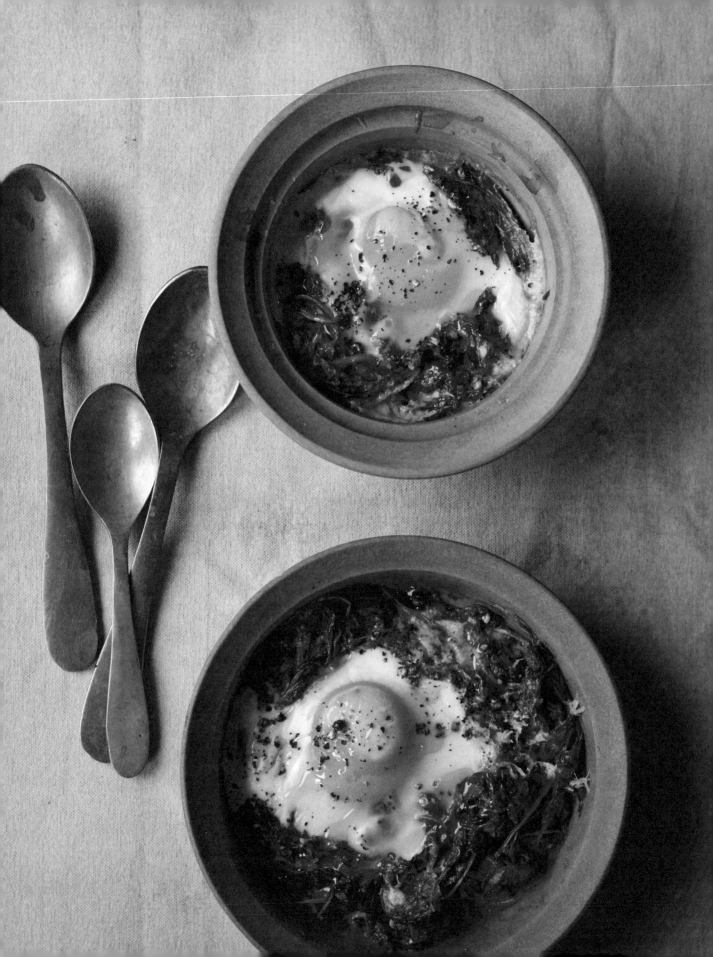

EASY EGGS in a CUP

SERVES 4, **VEG**, **GF**

This is a beautiful, quick dish that is good for breakfast or lunch. To avoid a watery end product, make sure the spinach is well dried prior to adding it to the sauté pan, because it will give up a lot of liquid as it cooks. A salad spinner is best for drying spinach quickly and efficiently. For a time-saver, buy prewashed, organic bagged spinach from the market.

1 tablespoon extra-virgin olive oil, plus more for oiling ramekins

Pinch of crushed red pepper flakes

½ cup finely diced onion

1 garlic clove, pressed and allowed to sit for 10 minutes

4 cups (about 6 ounces) tightly packed baby spinach

Sea salt

Pinch of freshly grated nutmeg

¼ cup freshly grated Parmesan cheese

4 eggs

Pinch of freshly ground black pepper

1. Preheat the oven to 375°F.

2. Heat the olive oil in a sauté pan over medium heat, then add the red pepper flakes and onion and sauté until the onion is translucent, about 3 minutes. Stir in the garlic and sauté for an additional 30 seconds, then stir in the spinach and a pinch of salt and cook until the spinach is wilted and tender, about another 30 seconds. Remove from the heat and stir in the nutmeg.

3. Lightly grease 4 small ramekins with olive oil. For each ramekin, spoon in one-fourth of the spinach mixture, then sprinkle on 1 tablespoon of the cheese. Gently crack 1 egg on top of the cheese, then sprinkle with pepper and a pinch of salt.

4. Bake for 12 to 14 minutes, until very little liquid remains.

5. Let cool for 3 minutes, then run a knife or an offset spatula around the inside edge of each ramekin to loosen the egg. Using your knife or spatula to help support the eggs, carefully transfer to a plate and serve immediately.

TOFU and BROCCOLI STIR-FRY

SERVES 4, **V**, **GF**

This simple stir-fried preparation of broccoli and tofu is an easy, satisfying main course. The drier the slices of tofu, the quicker they will sauté to a light golden color with a pleasantly chewy texture, contrasting nicely with the bright green, crisp-tender broccoli and the softer mushrooms, which absorb the richly flavored sauce.

3 tablespoons grapeseed oil

1 (10-ounce) package extra-firm tofu, drained, thinly sliced, and dried between paper towels or dish towels

½ onion, sliced

4 ounces shiitake mushrooms, stemmed and thinly sliced

1 pound broccoli, cut into florets, stalks peeled and cut into ½-inch chunks

2 teaspoons grated peeled ginger

1 garlic clove, pressed and allowed to sit for 10 minutes

½ cup Ginger-Garlic Stir-Fry Sauce (page 268)

1 tablespoon toasted sesame seeds

1. Heat 1 tablespoon of the oil in a 12-inch skillet set over medium-high heat. Lay in half the tofu and pan-fry, turning once when golden, about 4 minutes per side. Remove the tofu to a plate, add another tablespoon of oil, and repeat with the remaining tofu.

2. Add the remaining tablespoon of oil to the hot pan, then add the onions and mushrooms. Stir-fry until browned in spots, about 3 minutes. Add the broccoli stalks, ginger, and garlic to the pan and cook for another 30 seconds. Add the broccoli florets and stir-fry for a minute more. Add 1 to 2 tablespoons of water if the pan is dry. Add the tofu and the sauce, stir to coat, and cook another 1 to 2 minutes to allow the sauce to thicken. Garnish with sesame seeds and serve hot.

ZA'ATAR-CRUSTED CHICKEN PAILLARD

SERVES 4, GF

Za'atar is an herb-and-spice blend popular throughout the Middle East. It includes sesame seeds, salt, dried sumac berries, and thyme or oregano, or both. Often made at home in the region, za'atar is available in gourmet and Middle Eastern grocery stores and online (from penzeys.com, for one). Try it sprinkled on warm bread with olive oil or on fish and vegetables. Here it gives a distinctive accent to a quick and simple preparation of chicken breast. Paillard, or pounded, chicken is very tender and takes no time to cook. The trick is to allow it to sear quickly. As with fish, do not overcook. The chicken is so thinly pounded that it requires only a few minutes in the skillet.

4 (6-ounce) skinless, boneless chicken breasts, pounded to ¼ inch thick

Sea salt and freshly ground black pepper, to taste

2 tablespoons za'atar spice blend

2 tablespoons extra-virgin olive oil

¼ cup chopped flat-leaf parsley

4 teaspoons lemon juice

1. Season the chicken on both sides with salt, pepper, and the za'atar spice blend. Press the spices into each side of the chicken to form a thin crust.

2. Heat the olive oil in a large skillet over medium heat. Place the chicken in the pan and cook for 1 to 2 minutes per side or until golden brown.

3. Sprinkle each piece of chicken with parsley and lemon juice and serve immediately.

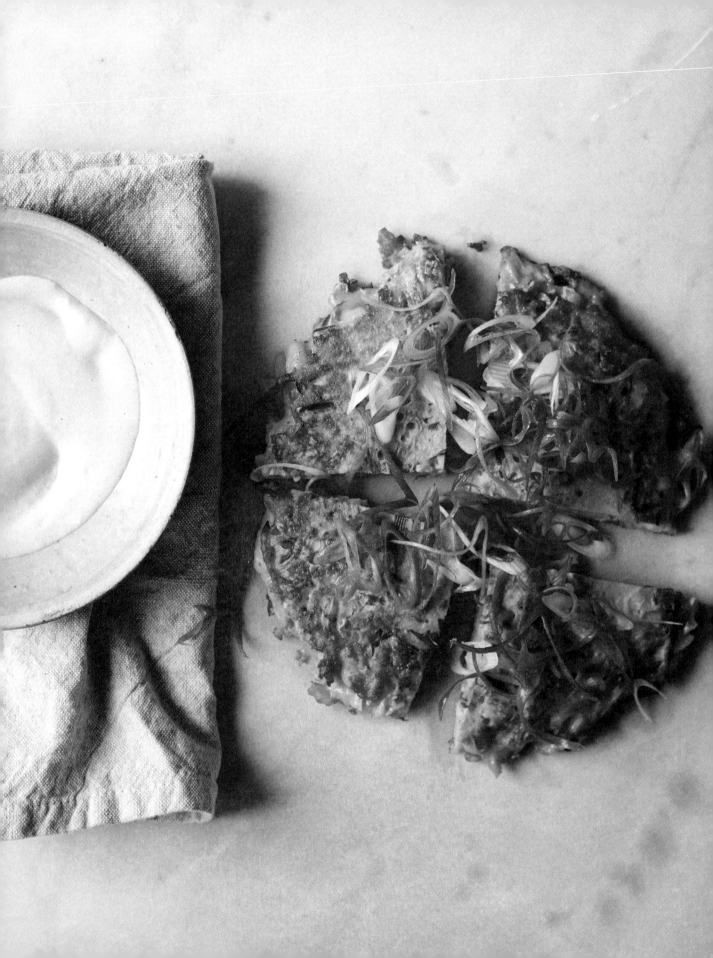

JAPANESE PANCAKE

MAKES TWO 6-INCH PANCAKES, **VEG***

This savory Japanese pancake, or *okonomiyaki* (*okonomi* means "what you like" and *yaki* means "grilled" or "cooked"), is made with cabbage and other vegetables and a variety of seafood and meats. In Japan, it's popular street food and is also served in restaurants, some of which let diners choose ingredients and cook the mixture on a personal hot plate. Too often, *okonomiyaki* is smothered with a thick, sweet sauce. I prefer this version, with a miso-mayo topping. I think you'll find it to be a great comfort food for either a main course or breakfast.

MISO MAYO

2 tablespoons mayonnaise

1½ teaspoons white (shiro) miso

1½ teaspoons unseasoned rice vinegar

PANCAKES

1 medium Napa cabbage, thinly sliced (about 4 cups)

½ medium sweet potato, peeled and grated

5 scallions, white and light green parts only, thinly sliced (reserve tops for garnish)

4 ounces raw shrimp, peeled, deveined, and coarsely chopped

¼ teaspoon sea salt

½ cup all-purpose flour

2 large eggs

¼ cup water or Dashi (page 266)

2 teaspoons low-sodium soy sauce

2 teaspoons unseasoned rice vinegar

2 teaspoons Sriracha sauce

½ teaspoon toasted sesame oil

2 teaspoons grapeseed oil

1. To make the Miso Mayo, combine all the ingredients in a small bowl, mix well, and set aside.

2. In a medium bowl, combine the cabbage, sweet potato, scallions, shrimp, and salt.

3. In separate large bowl, whisk together the flour, eggs, water or Dashi, soy sauce, rice vinegar, Sriracha sauce, and toasted sesame oil. Add the cabbage mixture to the batter and stir to combine.

4. Heat 1 teaspoon of the grapeseed oil in an 8-inch skillet over medium-low heat. Scoop half the batter into the center of the pan and flatten evenly out to

the edges so that the pancake is about ½ inch thick. Give the entire surface a few presses with a wide spatula, cover, and cook undisturbed for 5 to 6 minutes. Carefully turn over the pancake when it has a nice gold color and slides easily. Cook it for another 5 minutes, then remove the pancake to a plate. Add the remaining oil to the skillet and repeat with the remaining batter.

5. Cut the pancakes into wedges with a sharp knife or pizza cutter and serve with a drizzle of Miso Mayo. Garnish generously with scallion tops.

PURPLE PERUVIAN POTATO
and ZUCCHINI PANCAKES

SERVES 6, **VEG**

Purple potatoes are nutrient-dense with all their anthocyanin pigments, and they retain most of their color when cooked, so they look lovely with the green shredded zucchini and parsley in this recipe. I like to top these pancakes with a bit of smoked salmon, sablefish, or trout. Try them for breakfast.

½ pound purple Peruvian potatoes, peeled and grated

1 small zucchini, finely grated

½ small onion, grated

2 eggs, beaten

½ teaspoon sea salt

¼ teaspoon freshly ground black pepper

⅛ teaspoon freshly grated nutmeg

¼ cup tightly packed flat-leaf parsley leaves, finely chopped

1 tablespoon all-purpose flour

4 teaspoons grapeseed oil

Plain Greek yogurt

1. Put the potato, zucchini, and onion in a colander and press gently to squeeze out excess moisture.

2. Put the eggs, salt, pepper, and nutmeg in a large bowl and whisk to combine. Add the grated vegetables, parsley, and flour and stir with a spatula to combine.

3. Heat the grapeseed oil in a large skillet over medium heat. Spoon the mixture into the skillet by the heaping tablespoonful, then flatten with the back of the spoon.

4. Cook until golden brown on both sides, about 2 minutes per side. Transfer to a platter, keeping the pancakes in a single layer. Serve hot or warm with a dollop of Greek yogurt.

VARIATIONS: For extra protein, top the pancakes with smoked salmon, sablefish, trout, or a poached egg.

RED THAI CURRY

SERVES 4, **GF**

Despite the long ingredient list, this curry comes together very quickly. Tofu is the protein called for here, but as variations, salmon, shrimp, and chicken all work well. (In fact, this is a surefire way to poach salmon without overcooking.) The lime zest adds a distinctive Thai flavor. Serve with rice or rice noodles to sop up the curry sauce.

2 tablespoons grapeseed oil

1 tablespoon minced peeled ginger

3 garlic cloves, pressed and allowed to sit for 10 minutes

1½ tablespoons Thai red curry paste

2 carrots, peeled and sliced on the bias

1 small Yukon gold potato, diced into ½-inch cubes

1 red bell pepper, seeded and diced into ½-inch pieces

2 (16-ounce) cans light coconut milk

2 tablespoons fish sauce

1 pound broccoli florets

8 ounces extra-firm tofu, cut into ¾-inch cubes

2 teaspoons grated lime zest

1 tablespoon lime juice

½ teaspoon grade B maple syrup

4 scallions, white and light green parts only, thinly sliced on the bias

¼ cup packed fresh cilantro leaves, coarsely chopped

Lime wedges

1. Heat the oil in a large wide pan over medium heat. Add the ginger, garlic, and red curry paste, cook for 45 seconds, then add the carrots and sauté for 3 minutes.

2. Add the potatoes and peppers, stir to coat, and sauté for 2 minutes. Stir in the coconut milk, 1 cup of water, and the fish sauce and bring to a simmer. Cook, stirring occasionally, until the liquid is thickened and slightly reduced and the potatoes are just tender, about 8 minutes. Add the broccoli and tofu and cook, covered, until the broccoli is crisp-tender and the tofu is heated through, about 2 minutes.

3. Remove from the heat and stir in the lime zest, lime juice, and maple syrup. Top each portion with scallions, chopped cilantro, and a lime wedge.

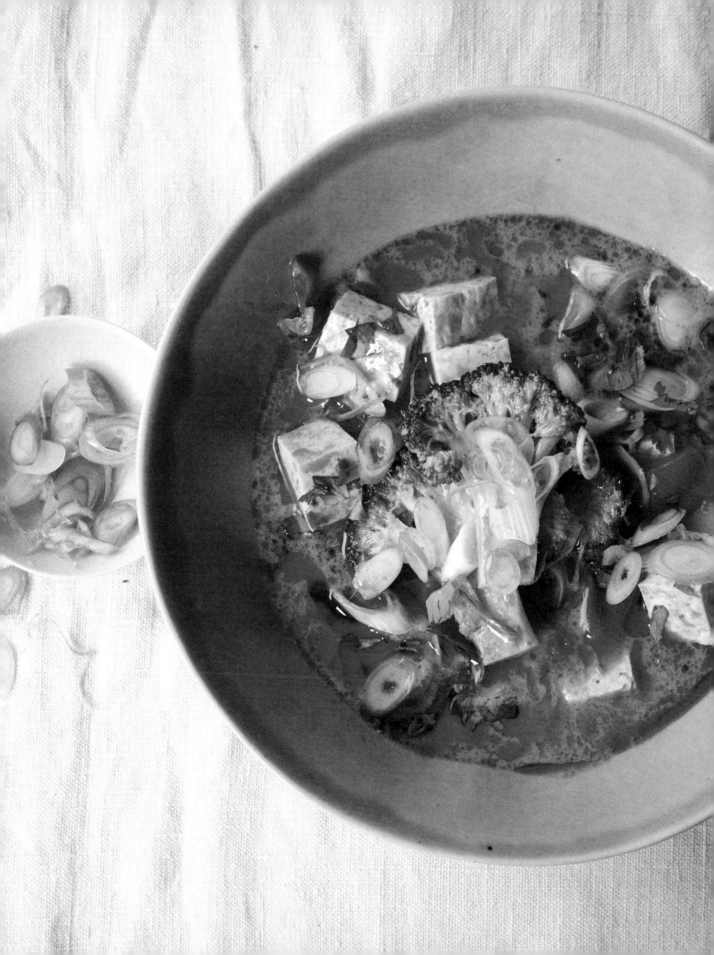

VARIATIONS:

Salmon: Cut ¾ pound skinless salmon fillet into ¾-inch cubes and add at the same time as the broccoli.

Shrimp: Add 16 peeled and deveined shrimp when the potatoes are tender and cook for 1 minute. Add the broccoli, cover, and cook for another 2 minutes.

Chicken: Add ½ pound thinly sliced chicken with the ginger and garlic. Cook and remove to a plate. Add back with the broccoli.

YUCATÁN BLACK BEAN and SWEET POTATO TOSTADAS

SERVES 4, **VEG**

This recipe comes together easily and is tremendously satisfying with the crisp tortilla, hearty black beans, sweet potatoes, crunchy cabbage slaw, and pumpkin seeds that pop as you bite them. This was inspired by the recipe for an open-faced enchilada from *Rebar: Modern Food Cookbook*. According to one story, the owners of the Rebar restaurant in Victoria, British Columbia, tried to take the popular dish off the menu, but customers wouldn't let them.

CABBAGE SLAW

2 tablespoons lime juice

2 tablespoons extra-virgin olive oil

½ teaspoon grade B maple syrup

¼ teaspoon sea salt

½ medium head red cabbage, thinly sliced (about 3 cups)

1 tablespoon minced seeded jalapeño pepper

¼ cup roughly chopped fresh cilantro leaves

FILLING

2 tablespoons extra-virgin olive oil

¼ cup finely chopped onion

½ teaspoon plus a pinch of sea salt, or more to taste

2 garlic cloves, pressed and allowed to sit for 10 minutes

1 medium sweet potato, peeled and cut into ¼-inch cubes

1 teaspoon chili powder

½ teaspoon ground cumin

¼ teaspoon ground cinnamon

¼ teaspoon cayenne pepper

1 (15-ounce) can black beans, rinsed and drained

1 tablespoon lime juice, or more to taste

TORTILLAS

4 corn tortillas

1 avocado, mashed with a fork

1 tablespoon toasted pumpkin seeds (page 274) (optional)

2 tablespoons crumbled queso fresco (optional)

1. Preheat the oven to 350°F.

2. In a medium bowl, whisk together the lime juice, olive oil, maple syrup, and ¼ teaspoon salt. Add the cabbage and jalapeño and toss to coat. Add the cilantro and toss again. Set aside.

3. Heat the oil in a medium pan over medium-high heat. Add the onion and a pinch of salt and sauté for 3 minutes. Add the garlic and sauté for 45 seconds. Add the sweet potatoes, spices, and the remaining ½ teaspoon of salt and sauté for 6 minutes or until the potatoes are just tender. Stir in the beans and cook for 3 minutes. Remove the pan from the heat and add the lime juice. Taste and adjust the seasoning with more lime juice or salt, if necessary.

4. Place the tortillas on a cookie sheet and bake for 8 minutes or until just crisp.

5. To assemble the tostadas, spread a spoonful of avocado on each tortilla and top with the black bean–sweet potato mixture and then the cabbage slaw. Sprinkle with pumpkin seeds and queso fresco, if desired.

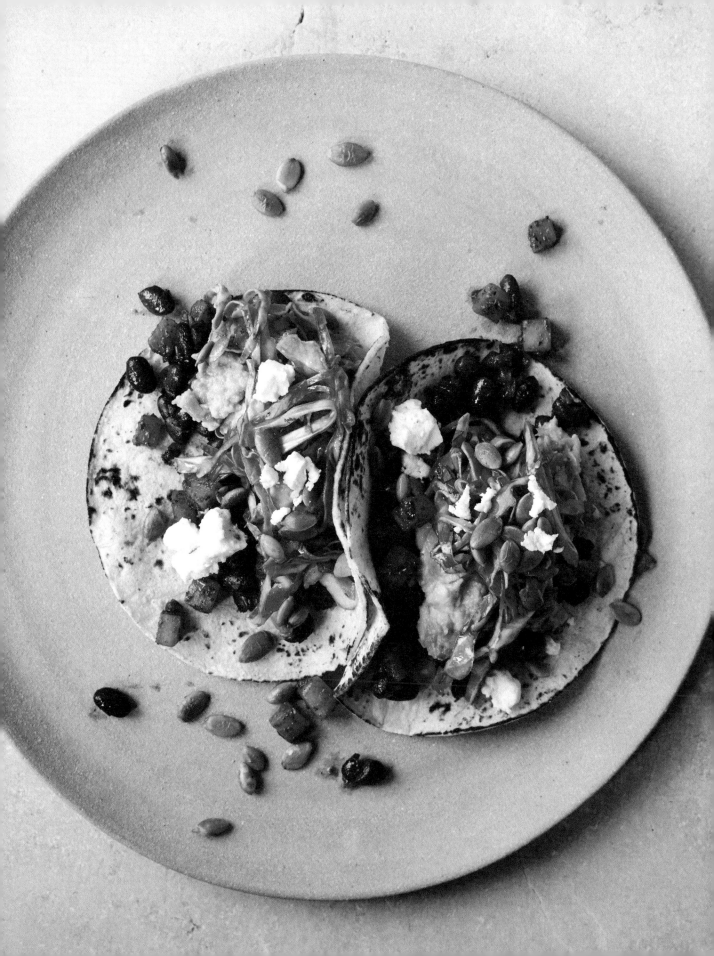

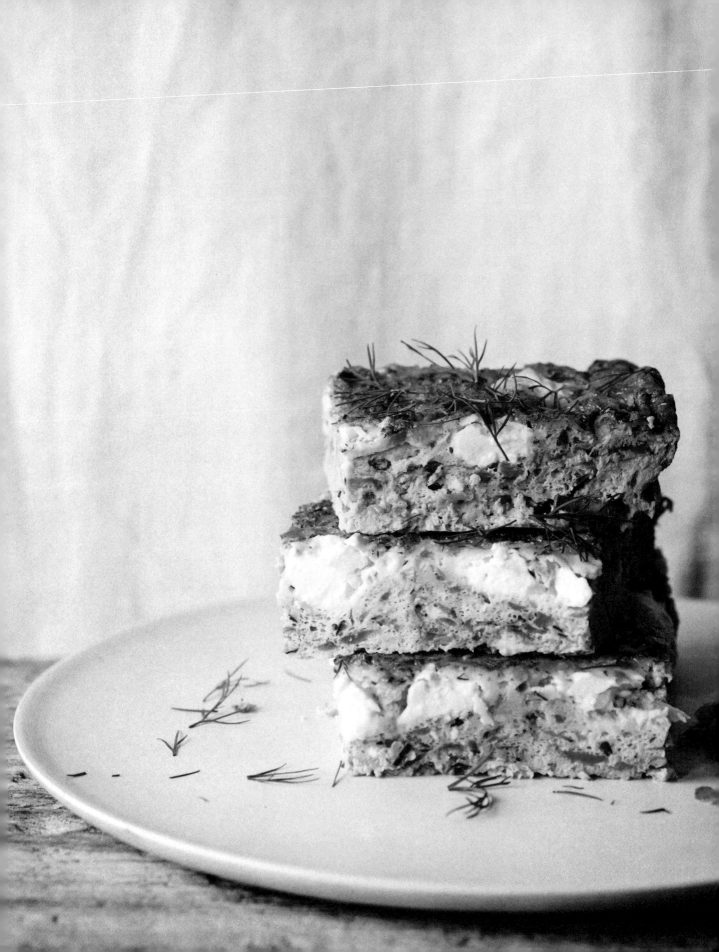

VEGETABLE FRITTATA
with FETA and DILL

SERVES 6, **VEG**

A frittata is an Italian egg cake in which various ingredients, from vegetables to meat to pasta, are incorporated into beaten eggs and baked. This vegetarian version has onion, carrot, and zucchini livened up with dill weed and crumbled feta cheese. It can be paired with a salad for a light lunch and also makes a good breakfast dish.

2 tablespoons extra-virgin olive oil

½ onion, diced

½ teaspoon plus 3 pinches of sea salt

1 carrot, peeled and shredded

1 zucchini, shredded

8 large eggs

¾ teaspoon dried dill

¼ teaspoon freshly ground black pepper

6 tablespoons crumbled feta

1. Preheat the oven to 350°F.

2. Using ½ tablespoon of the olive oil, grease an 8-by-8-inch glass or ceramic baking dish.

3. In a medium sauté pan, heat the remaining oil over medium-high heat. Add the onions and a pinch of salt. Stir and cook for about 4 minutes. Add the carrots and another pinch of salt. Stir and cook for about a minute. Add the zucchini and a third pinch of salt. Stir and cook for another 2 minutes. Put the vegetables into the greased pan and set aside.

4. Whisk together the eggs, 1 tablespoon of water, dill, the remaining ½ teaspoon of salt, and pepper. Pour over the vegetables, then sprinkle the feta over the top.

5. Bake for about 20 minutes or until the center is just set.

6. Remove from the oven, cool for a few minutes, then cut into squares. Serve hot or at room temperature.

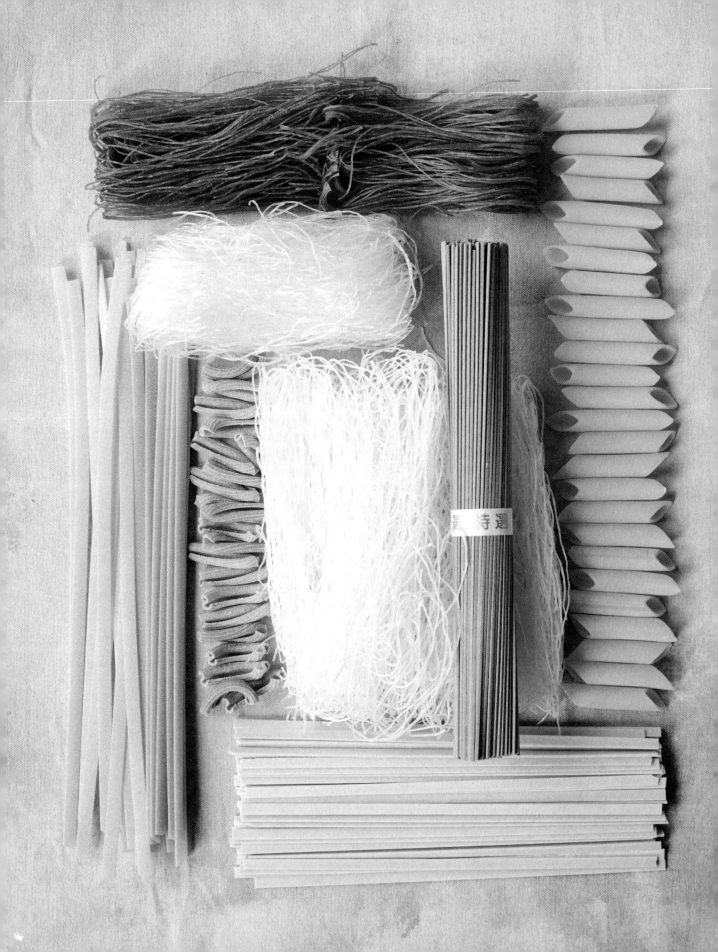

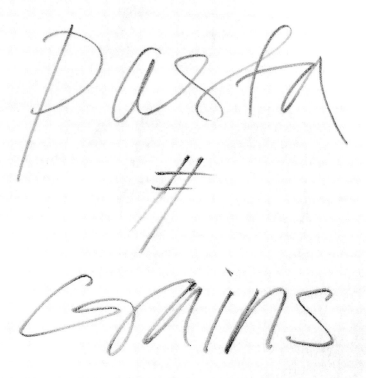

Pasta & Grains

Pasta and grains have fallen into disfavor in recent years, caught up in a rising tide of carbohydrate phobia and concerns about glycemic load and gluten sensitivity. Truly whole grains (or grains cracked into a few big pieces) are nutrient-rich foods that are digested slowly without causing spikes in blood sugar or insulin resistance. Despite labels to the contrary, whole-wheat flour and most whole-wheat breads are not whole-grain foods; from the point of view of glycemic load, they are little different from white flour and white bread. Some grains used in this book, like spelt and farro, have a lower gluten content than modern wheat, and good gluten-free pasta is available. When it comes to pasta, portion size is key. In short, I believe that true whole grains and moderate amounts of pasta are consistent with healthy eating and the principles of the Anti-Inflammatory Diet.

Recipes marked **veg** are vegetarian, those marked **v** are vegan, and those marked **gf** are gluten-free. The symbols **veg***, **v***, and **gf*** indicate recipes that can be modified to be vegetarian, vegan, or gluten-free by substituting or omitting specific ingredients.

LINGUINE with CLAMS

SERVES 6

Linguine alle vongole is a classic Italian seafood-and-pasta dish in which clams in their shells are quickly cooked in a covered pot with olive oil, a lot of garlic, red pepper flakes, and white wine. (I use white vermouth for extra flavor.) The clams steam quickly in their own juice and are then poured over cooked linguine—shells, broth, and all— and topped with a quantity of chopped fresh flat-leaf parsley. Serve it all in a large platter for a dramatic presentation, providing plenty of paper towels and bowls for discarded shells. You can omit the pasta and let your guests dip hunks of rustic bread into the flavorful broth or just slurp it up with a spoon. It is usually not necessary to add salt to this dish; the clam juice will be salty enough on its own.

2 pounds littleneck or butter clams, scrubbed

Sea salt

1 pound dried linguine

¼ cup extra-virgin olive oil

½ cup dry (white) vermouth

6 garlic cloves, pressed and allowed to sit for 10 minutes

1 teaspoon crushed red pepper flakes

½ cup chopped fresh flat-leaf parsley leaves

1. Rinse clams well.

2. Bring a large pot of salted water to a boil. Add the linguine and cook until al dente.

3. Meanwhile, heat the oil in a deep skillet over high heat. Add the clams, vermouth, garlic, and red pepper flakes. Cover and steam the clams until most of them open, about 6 to 7 minutes (discard the unopened clams). Remove from the heat.

4. Drain the pasta, place it in a deep platter, and toss it with a ladleful of the clam broth.

5. Pour the clams and most of the remaining broth over the pasta and top with the parsley. Serve at once.

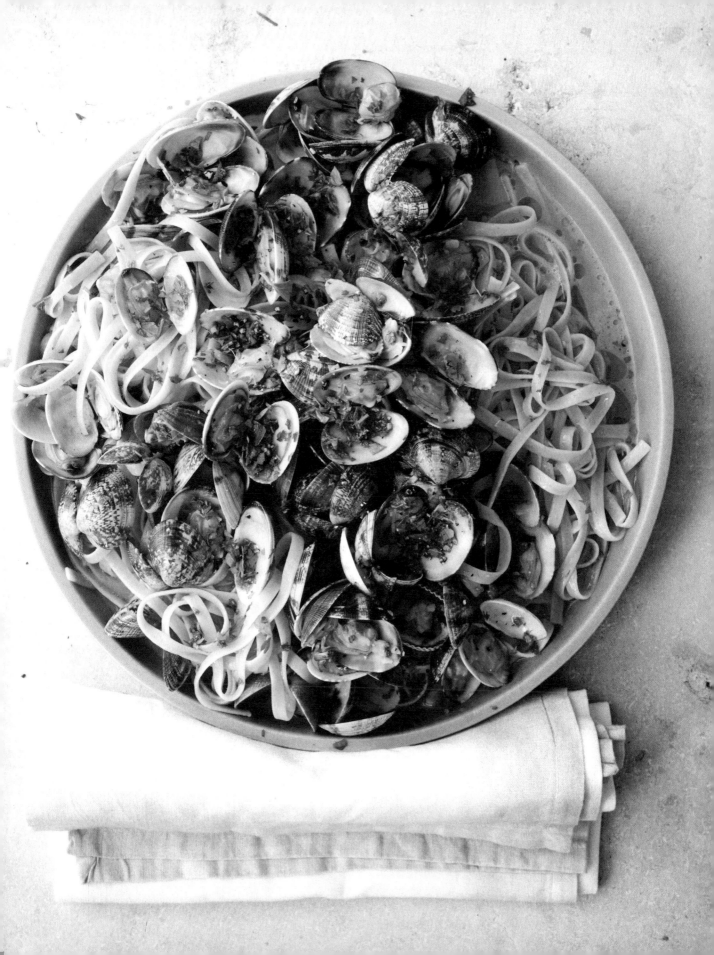

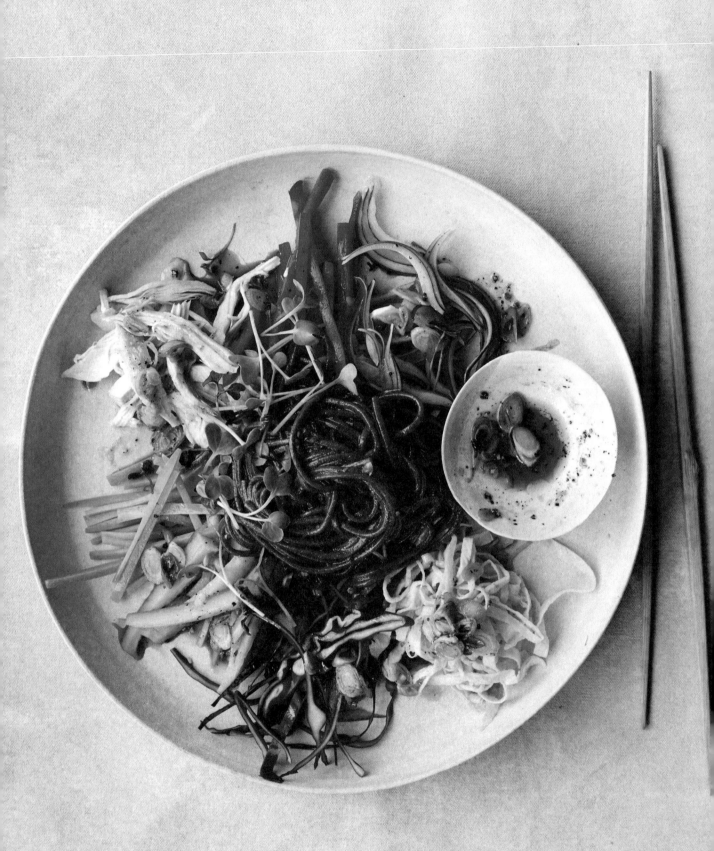

COLD BUCKWHEAT NOODLES with CHICKEN or TOFU and VEGETABLES

SERVES 4, **V***

I use Japanese soba noodles, made from a mixture of buckwheat and wheat, for this wonderful dish that can stand on its own for a light meal, even for breakfast. For a vegan version, omit the chicken or replace it with slices of packaged baked pressed tofu.

DRESSING

¼ cup low-sodium soy sauce

1¼ tablespoons evaporated cane sugar

2 tablespoons water

1 tablespoon mirin

2 tablespoons lime juice

2 teaspoons Sriracha or your favorite hot sauce, to taste

1 tablespoon toasted sesame oil

3 scallions, white and light green parts only, finely chopped

NOODLES

8 ounces buckwheat (soba) noodles

2 large red cabbage leaves, shredded

1 small red bell pepper, seeded and thinly sliced

1 carrot, peeled and julienned

1 cucumber, peeled, seeded, and julienned

1 small red onion, thinly sliced and soaked in ice water for 5 minutes

1 cup shredded cooked chicken or sliced baked pressed tofu

1½ cups radish sprouts

1. In a medium bowl, whisk together the dressing ingredients and reserve.

2. Bring a large pot of water to a boil and cook the noodles for 5 to 6 minutes, or until tender. Drain in a colander and rinse under cold water. Toss the noodles with half the dressing.

3. Arrange the vegetables and chicken or tofu on a large serving platter. Place the noodles in the middle and top with the radish sprouts. Just before serving, pour the remaining dressing over the noodles and vegetables and toss.

SPICED COUSCOUS
with SLIVERED ALMONDS

SERVES 6, **V**

This is super-fast and includes many warming anti-inflammatory spices. Citrus juice and zest really punch up the flavor, while the almonds add a nice crunch and the currants a pleasing chew. I came across a dish like this in Sicily that used pistachios instead of almonds.

3 tablespoons extra-virgin olive oil

½ onion, diced

¾ teaspoon plus a pinch of sea salt

¾ teaspoon ground cinnamon

¼ teaspoon ground cloves

¼ teaspoon ground nutmeg

1 cup couscous

¼ cup sliced almonds, toasted, plus more for garnish (page 274)

3 tablespoons currants

2 tablespoons orange juice

1½ teaspoons grated orange zest

2 teaspoons lemon juice

1. Heat the oil in a medium sauté pan over medium-high heat. Add the onions with a pinch of salt and sauté for about 6 minutes or until translucent and golden.

2. Add the rest of the salt, the cinnamon, cloves, and nutmeg and stir to combine. Add the couscous and toast, stirring, for about a minute. Add 1 cup of boiling water and stir until combined. Remove from the heat, cover, and let sit for 5 minutes.

3. Fluff with a fork, then fold in the almonds, currants, orange juice, orange zest, and lemon juice. Garnish with more almonds.

FORBIDDEN RICE with GINGER and LEMONGRASS

SERVES 4, **V, GF**

Forbidden rice, more commonly known as black or purple rice, comes in several varieties from Indonesia and Thailand. Much esteemed for its health benefits in China, where, supposedly, it was once forbidden to all but emperors, black rice is unusually high in antioxidants due to the large amount of anthocyanin pigments it contains (it has even more than blueberries). It's such a beauty—a whole grain that cooks in 20 minutes—it leaves brown rice in the dust, in my opinion. This is a simple recipe that will pair perfectly with every fish dish in the book.

2 (½-inch) slices unpeeled ginger

2 stalks lemongrass, cut into thirds, scored, and smashed

½ teaspoon sea salt

1 cup forbidden rice

1. Bring 2 cups of water, the sliced ginger, lemongrass, and salt to a boil, then stir in the rice.

2. Cover, lower the heat, and simmer for 20 minutes, then let stand covered for 10 more minutes. Check to see if the rice is tender. Remove the ginger slices and lemongrass and serve.

FARRO SALAD with MARINATED FETA, OLIVES, and PARSLEY

SERVES 4, **VEG**

Quick-cooking pearled farro is the chewy, nutty centerpiece of this novel riff on tabbouleh. The whole grain is mixed with a colorful assortment of chopped raw vegetables, seasoned with garlic and allspice, and dressed with olive oil and fresh lemon juice. The topping of marinated feta is a knockout, dramatically flavored with coriander, cumin, and za'atar (see page 175 for a description of that Middle Eastern mix of herbs and spices). You can chop the vegetables, parsley, and olives while the farro cooks.

FETA TOPPING

1 cup dry feta, crumbled

2 teaspoons za'atar

1 teaspoon ground coriander

½ teaspoon ground cumin

2 tablespoons extra-virgin olive oil

SALAD

1 cup pearled farro

1 small red bell pepper, seeded and diced

1 English cucumber, peeled, seeded, and diced

1 pint cherry tomatoes, halved

1 bunch fresh flat-leaf parsley, leaves picked and finely chopped

4 scallions, white and light green parts only, finely sliced

½ cup pitted and coarsely chopped Kalamata olives

½ teaspoon ground allspice

2 garlic cloves, pressed and allowed to sit for 10 minutes

2 tablespoons lemon juice

Sea salt and freshly ground black pepper, to taste

3 tablespoons extra-virgin olive oil

1. In a small bowl, combine the feta, za'atar, coriander, and cumin. Toss with 2 tablespoons of the olive oil.

2. Heat a medium saucepan over medium-high heat and add the farro. Dry toast it for 2 to 3 minutes, then pour in enough water to fill the pan halfway. Cover the pan partially with a lid and bring to a boil. Reduce the heat to medium-low and cook for 15 to 18 minutes until the farro is tender but al dente. Drain and let it cool. Transfer to a mixing bowl.

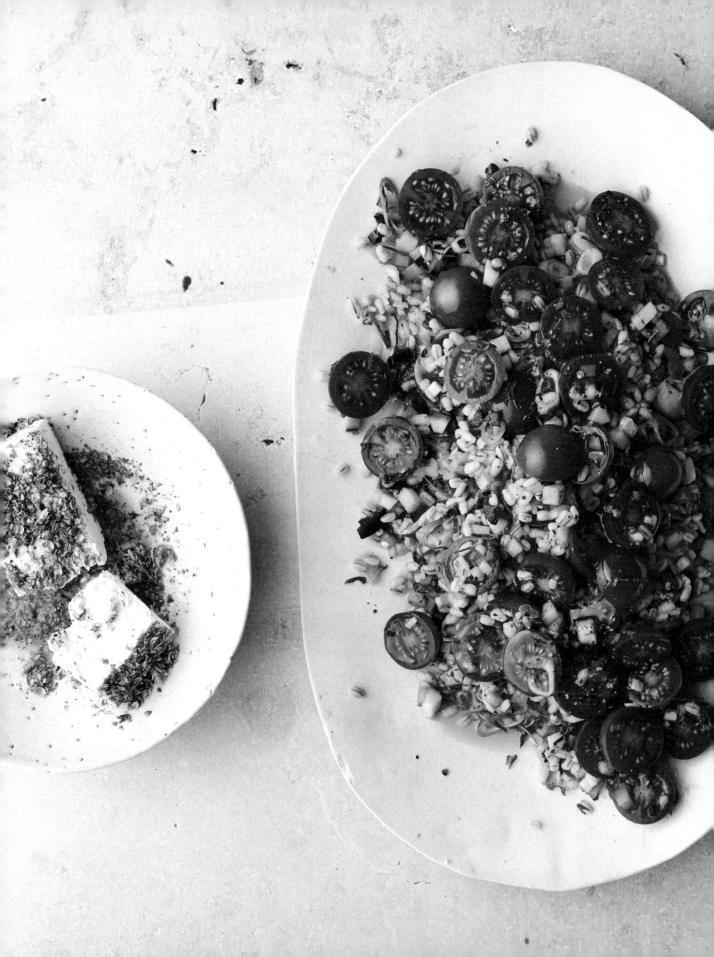

3. Add the bell pepper, cucumber, tomatoes, parsley, scallions, olives, and allspice. In a small bowl, whisk the garlic and lemon juice together and pour over the vegetables. Season the salad with a large pinch of both salt and black pepper and the remaining 3 tablespoons of oil. Gently toss until evenly dressed. Place in bowls and garnish each portion with the feta topping.

STIR-FRIED SWEET POTATO NOODLES
with PRAWNS and VEGETABLES

SERVES 4, **V***, **GF**

This recipe is based on a popular vegetarian dish in Korea prepared with chewy, transparent noodles made from sweet potato starch. These are gluten-free and lower in glycemic load than most pasta. The dried noodles are readily available online and in Asian grocery stores. Here they are quickly reconstituted in hot water, rinsed, mixed with a bit of toasted sesame oil, then added to stir-fried vegetables and a flavorful sauce. Koreans enjoy this both hot and cold as a side dish, but you can turn it into a more substantial main course by adding seafood or tofu. (Note: muscovado sugar is an unrefined brown sugar that's readily available at markets or online.)

8 ounces dried Korean sweet potato noodles

2 teaspoons toasted sesame oil

¼ cup low-sodium soy sauce

1 tablespoon (packed) muscovado sugar

1 tablespoon grapeseed oil

1 large carrot, peeled and cut in 2-inch matchsticks

1 onion, thinly sliced

¼ teaspoon freshly ground black pepper or crushed red pepper flakes to taste

Pinch of sea salt

8 ounces shiitake, stemmed and thinly sliced

2 garlic cloves, pressed and allowed to sit for 10 minutes

6 ounces raw peeled and deveined prawns or baked pressed tofu, sliced (optional)

6 ounces baby spinach

3 scallions, white and light green parts only, thinly sliced

1 tablespoon toasted sesame seeds

1. Bring a large pot of water to a boil. Add the noodles, stir to separate them, and cook for about 4 to 5 minutes. Drain in a colander and rinse under cold water. Using scissors, cut the noodles into 6- to 8-inch lengths. With the noodles still in the colander, drizzle with the sesame oil and toss to coat. Set aside.

2. In a small bowl, mix the soy sauce and sugar together until the sugar dissolves. Set aside.

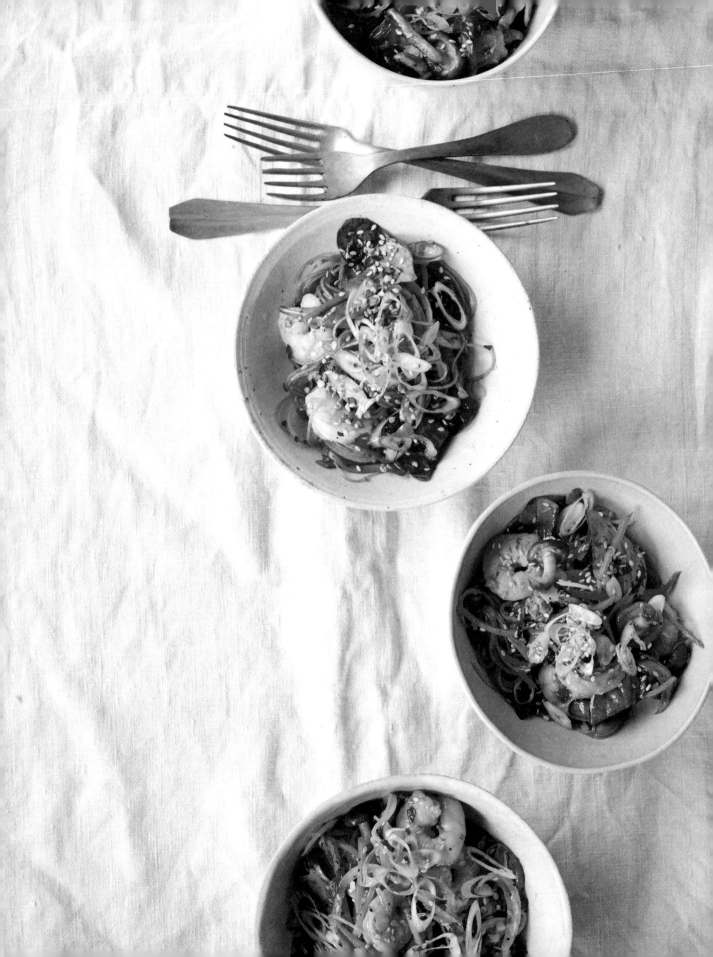

3. Heat the grapeseed oil in a large nonstick skillet over medium heat. Add the carrots, onions, black pepper, and a pinch of salt. Cook, stirring occasionally, until the onion has softened, about 4 minutes. Add the mushrooms and garlic (and prawns or tofu) and cook, stirring occasionally, until the mushrooms are cooked through, about 5 minutes. Add the noodles and soy sauce mixture and toss until heated through, about 2 minutes. Add the spinach and, using tongs, toss to combine. Cook until the spinach is wilted, about 1 minute more.

4. Transfer to a serving platter and sprinkle with the scallions and sesame seeds. Serve hot or at room temperature.

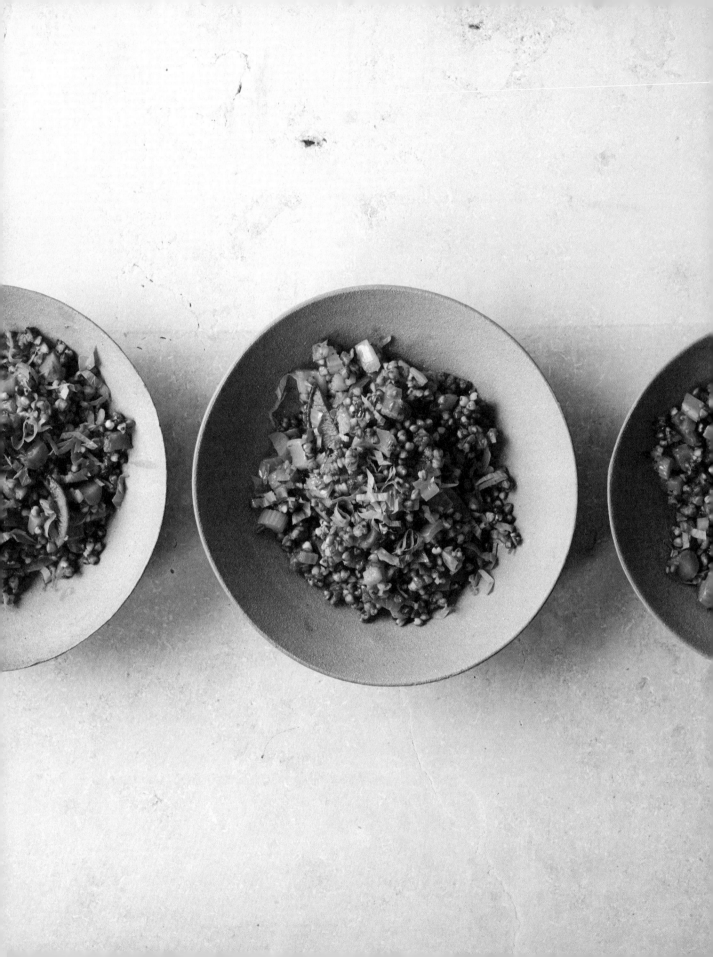

KASHA with VEGETABLES

SERVES 4, **V, GF**

Kasha is a sort of porridge made from toasted buckwheat groats—that is, the hulled kernels of buckwheat, a grainlike seed unrelated to wheat and gluten-free. Kasha is a popular food in Russia and Poland and was brought to the United States by Jewish immigrants from those countries in the early years of the twentieth century. Kasha is richly aromatic with a distinctive, nutty taste. It cooks quickly and makes an unusual and nutritious whole-grain preparation that seems most suited to fall and winter meals. Dried, reconstituted shiitake mushrooms and their soaking liquid greatly enhance the flavor of the dish.

2 ounces dried shiitake mushrooms

1 tablespoon extra-virgin olive oil

1 onion, coarsely chopped

1 large carrot, peeled and sliced

1 celery stalk, sliced

1 cup toasted buckwheat groats (kasha)

½ teaspoon sea salt

Freshly ground black pepper, to taste

1 cup water or vegetable broth

1 tablespoon finely chopped fresh flat-leaf parsley leaves

1. Rinse the mushrooms in cold water, place them in a bowl with 1 cup of warm water, and soak until the mushroom caps are soft. (Alternatively, you can place the mushrooms in a bowl with the water and microwave for 1 minute.) Drain and save the soaking water. Discard the tough stems and slice the caps ¼ inch thick. Set aside.

2. Heat the olive oil in a medium pot over medium-high heat. Add the onion, carrot, and celery and sauté for 2 minutes. Add the kasha and sauté for 1 minute more. Add the sliced mushrooms, salt, black pepper, 1 cup of the reserved mushroom liquid, and 1 cup of water or broth. Bring to a boil, cover, and simmer until the liquid is absorbed, about 15 minutes.

3. Fluff the mixture with a fork. Taste and adjust with salt or pepper, if necessary. Garnish with parsley and serve.

MUSHROOM QUINOA PILAF

SERVES 6, **V***, **GF**

Quick-cooking quinoa allows you to make a hearty mushroom pilaf in a fraction of the time that it takes to prepare a rice pilaf. Use several types of mushrooms, including any wild ones that are available. You will be tempted to stir the mushrooms around in the pan from the start, but the key here is to allow the cooking process to begin without moving them so that they can caramelize a bit, bringing out their earthy flavors and meaty texture.

3 tablespoons extra-virgin olive oil

1 large shallot, finely chopped

½ teaspoon plus a pinch of sea salt

1 cup quinoa, rinsed

1¾ cups Quick Vegetable Stock (page 266) or store-bought vegetable broth, chicken broth, or water

1 pound fresh mushrooms (cremini, shiitake, oyster, maitake, or others), stemmed and cut into ¼-inch slices

¼ teaspoon freshly ground black pepper

1 tablespoon chopped fresh thyme, or 1 teaspoon dried thyme

¼ cup finely chopped fresh flat-leaf parsley leaves

1. Heat 1 tablespoon of the oil in a medium pot over medium heat. Add the shallots and a pinch of salt. Sauté for 1 minute, until shallots are translucent. Add the quinoa to the pan and toast for a minute, stirring frequently. Add the stock and ¼ teaspoon of the salt. Bring to a boil, then reduce the heat to medium-low and cover. Let the quinoa simmer for 10 to 15 minutes. When the liquid is absorbed, remove from the heat and fluff with a fork.

2. Meanwhile, in a large skillet, heat 1 tablespoon of the remaining oil over medium-high heat. Add half the mushrooms in a single layer, half the pepper, and half the remaining salt. Cook without stirring until the mushrooms begin to brown on the bottom, about 2 minutes. Add half the thyme, stir, and continue to cook until well browned, about 5 minutes more. Remove cooked mushrooms to a serving bowl. Repeat with the remaining oil, raw mushrooms, pepper, salt, and thyme, and add this batch to the first one.

3. Fold the quinoa and parsley into the mushrooms and serve immediately.

PAPPARDELLE with ARUGULA WALNUT PESTO

SERVES 8, **VEG**

A variation on basil pesto, this bright green, vitamin- and mineral-packed sauce makes a delicious topping for wide, flat pasta. *Pappardelle* comes from an Italian verb meaning "to gobble up." (Try to resist that temptation.) Use fettuccine if you can't find pappardelle.

2 garlic cloves, pressed and allowed to sit for 10 minutes

3 loosely packed cups (about 4 ounces) baby arugula

1 loosely packed cup fresh basil leaves

¼ cup raw walnuts, toasted (page 274)

1 tablespoon lemon juice, or more to taste

⅓ cup extra-virgin olive oil

Sea salt

Freshly ground black pepper, to taste

1 pound dried pappardelle

¾ cup freshly grated Parmesan cheese, plus more for serving

1. Put the first eight ingredients in a food processor and process until smooth. Taste and adjust with more lemon juice, salt, and pepper, if necessary. Put the mixture in a medium bowl.

2. Bring a large pot of salted water to the boil. Add the pasta and cook according to the package directions until al dente.

3. Just before the pasta is done, remove 2 tablespoons of the pasta water and add it to the pesto. Add the cheese and mix well.

4. Drain the pasta and toss it with the pesto mixture. Serve with extra Parmesan cheese on the side.

QUICK BISON BOLOGNESE

SERVES 4, GF

Bolognese means "in the style of Bologna," the Italian city in the fertile Po valley renowned for cuisine that makes liberal use of meats and cheeses. A classic dish from the region is *ragù*, a rich sauce of meat, often flavored with tomatoes, served over pasta. This quick version with bison is hearty and delicious. Served with a simple salad, it makes a satisfying meal.

2 tablespoons extra-virgin olive oil

1 medium onion, finely chopped

2 stalks celery, finely chopped

1 carrot, peeled and finely chopped

¼ teaspoon crushed red pepper flakes

1 teaspoon sea salt, plus more to taste

1 pound ground bison

¼ teaspoon freshly ground black pepper, plus more to taste

1 tablespoon tomato paste

⅓ cup dry red wine

1 (28-ounce) can crushed tomatoes

⅛ teaspoon ground cinnamon

1 pound dried tagliatelle or fettuccine

¼ cup chopped fresh flat-leaf parsley leaves

Grated Parmesan cheese, for serving

1. Heat the oil in a large Dutch oven over medium-high heat. Add the onion, celery, carrot, red pepper flakes, and ¼ teaspoon of the salt. Sauté the vegetables until soft and just turning golden brown, about 5 minutes.

2. Add the bison, ½ teaspoon of the salt, and the pepper. Brown the bison, breaking it up with the back of a spoon, for 5 minutes. Add the tomato paste and mix it into the vegetables and meat. Pour in the wine and scrape the bottom of the pan with a wooden spoon to lift any browned bits. Cook, uncovered, until the wine has nearly evaporated. Add the tomatoes, the remaining ¼ teaspoon salt, and the cinnamon.

3. Allow the sauce to simmer uncovered for 15 to 20 minutes. Taste and adjust the seasoning with more salt or pepper, if necessary.

4. Bring a large pot of salted water to the boil. Add the pasta and cook according to the package directions until al dente. Transfer the pasta to a large serving bowl and mix in a ladle of the sauce to coat the pasta. Ladle the rest of the sauce on top and sprinkle with parsley. Serve immediately with Parmesan cheese on the side.

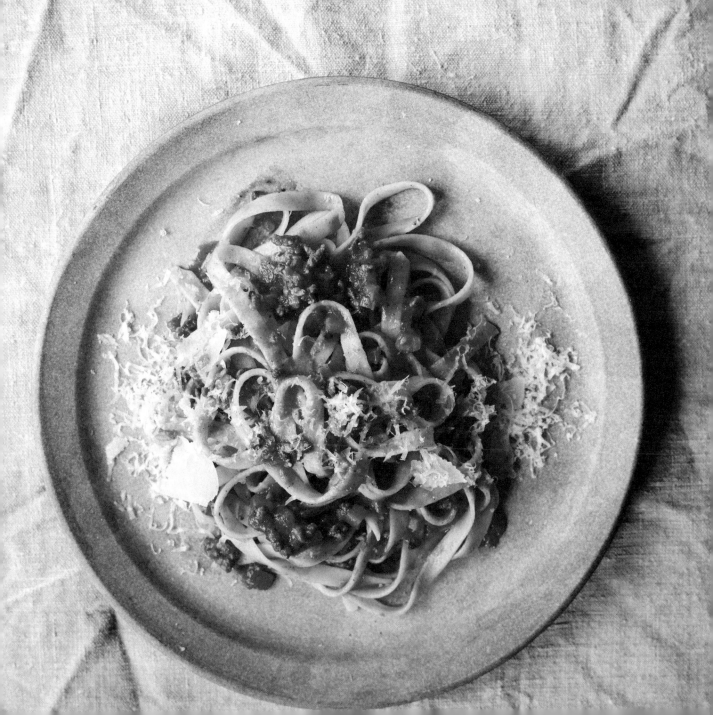

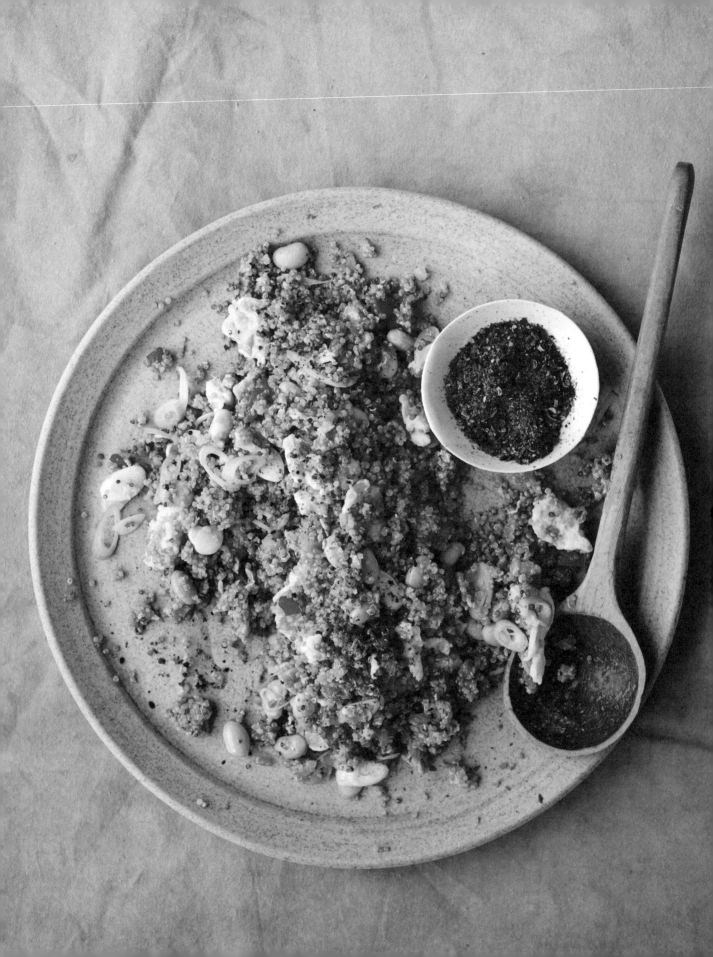

QUINOA FRIED "RICE"

SERVES 6, **VEG**, **V***, **GF**

Chinese fried rice requires you to prepare rice in advance and then chill it. Quick-cooking quinoa allows you to put together a similar grain-and-vegetable dish in a fraction of the time. Many variations are possible; use the ingredients you have on hand to get a balance of colors, textures, and flavors. This even works for breakfast.

1¾ cups Quick Vegetable Stock (page 266) or store-bought broth or water

¼ teaspoon sea salt

1 cup quinoa, rinsed

3 tablespoons grapeseed oil

1 onion, diced

⅓ cup seeded, diced red bell pepper

1 tablespoon low-sodium soy sauce

2 large eggs

1 cup baby spinach

¼ cup shelled edamame (green soybeans)

2 scallions, white and light green parts only, thinly sliced

2 teaspoons toasted sesame oil

shichimi (page 273) (optional)

1. In a medium pot, bring the broth or water and salt to a boil. Add the quinoa, stir, cover, and reduce the heat to medium-low. Let the quinoa cook for 10 to 15 minutes, stirring once halfway through, until it is just tender and the liquid is absorbed. Remove from the heat and fluff with a fork.

2. Heat the oil in a large skillet over medium-high heat. Add the onions and sauté until slightly golden, about 3 to 4 minutes. Stir in the red pepper and continue to cook another minute. Stir in the quinoa, then add the soy sauce and stir until well combined.

3. Push the quinoa mixture aside so that the bottom of pan is exposed. Break the eggs into the middle and scramble them with a thin spatula until they are set, about 2 minutes.

4. Reincorporate the quinoa and stir in the spinach, edamame, and scallions. Remove from the heat, drizzle with sesame oil and sprinkle shichimi on top, and serve hot.

VARIATIONS: You can substitute carrots for peppers, or peas for edamame. Add chunks or strips of baked pressed tofu in place of or in addition to the eggs.

QUINOA with DATES, OLIVES, ARUGULA, and SPEARMINT

SERVES 4, **V, GF**

Here is a tabbouleh-like grain salad made with quick-cooking quinoa, greens, and a zesty dressing, with the unexpected chewy sweetness of chopped dates.

1¾ cups Quick Vegetable Stock (page 266) or store-bought vegetable broth or water

½ teaspoon sea salt, or more to taste

1 cup quinoa, rinsed

1 teaspoon grated lemon zest

1 tablespoon lemon juice, or more to taste

¼ teaspoon freshly ground black pepper

2 tablespoons extra-virgin olive oil

1 cup arugula

12 Kalamata olives, pitted and sliced

2 tablespoons chopped dates

2 tablespoons finely chopped fresh flat-leaf parsley leaves

2 tablespoons finely chopped fresh spearmint

1. In a small saucepan, bring the broth and ¼ teaspoon of the salt to a boil over high heat. Add the quinoa, stir, cover, and reduce the heat to medium-low. Let the quinoa cook for 10 to 15 minutes (stirring once halfway through) until it is just tender and the liquid is absorbed. Remove from the heat and fluff with a fork.

2. In a large bowl, mix together the lemon zest, lemon juice, remaining ¼ teaspoon salt, pepper, and olive oil. Add the quinoa, arugula, olives, dates, parsley, and spearmint and toss well to combine. Taste and adjust the seasoning with more lemon juice, salt, or pepper, if necessary. Serve warm or at room temperature.

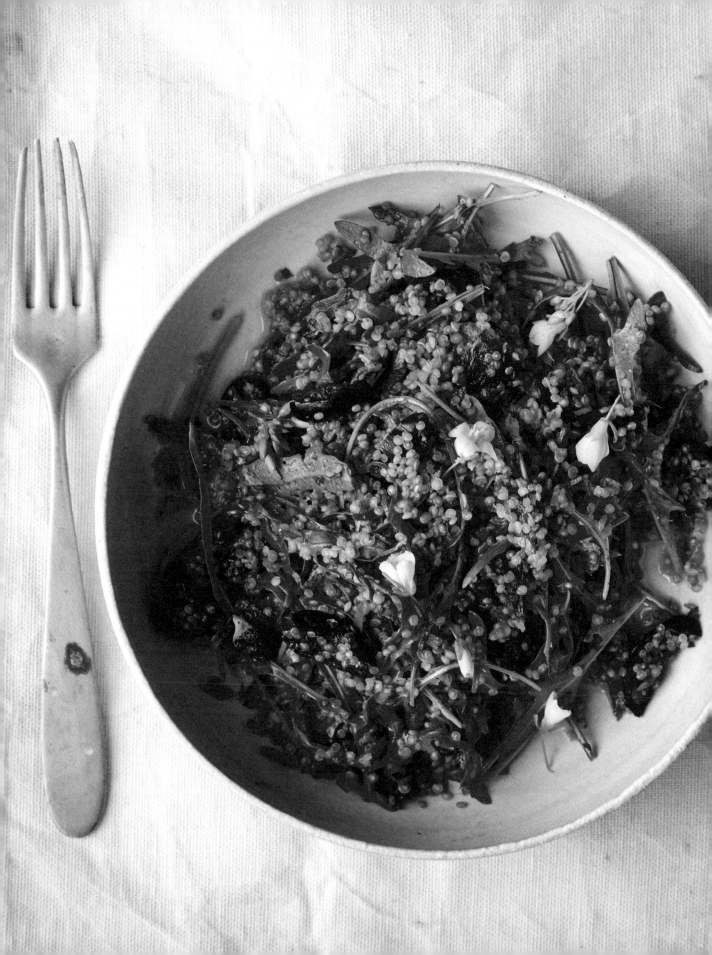

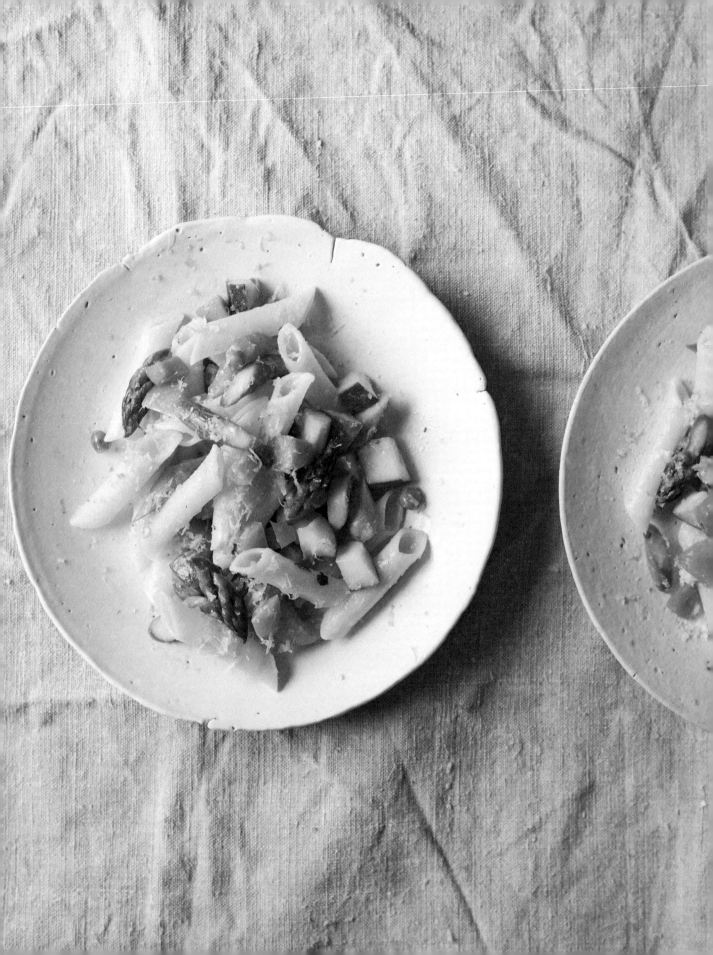

PASTA PRIMAVERA

SERVES 6, **VEG**

Primavera is Italian for "spring," and this classic pasta dish should suggest that season with its bright and crisp mix of fresh vegetables in a simple olive oil and garlic sauce accented with fresh herbs and lemon juice. Restaurant versions heavy with cream and butter miss the point. Be careful not to overcook the vegetables; you want them just crisp-tender, not soft.

1 pound dried penne

¼ cup extra-virgin olive oil

3 garlic cloves, pressed and left to sit for 10 minutes

Crushed red pepper flakes (optional)

1 large carrot, peeled and cut into ½-inch dice

1 large zucchini, cut into ½-inch dice

1 red bell pepper, seeded and cut into ½-inch dice

½ pound asparagus, trimmed and cut on the bias into ½-inch pieces

1½ cups frozen sweet peas, thawed

½ teaspoon sea salt

1 tablespoon lemon juice

1 cup finely grated Parmesan cheese

3 tablespoons finely chopped fresh flat-leaf parsley leaves

1. Bring 4 quarts of salted water to a boil in a large pot, add the penne, and cook according to package directions until the pasta is al dente. Have 6 warmed pasta bowls ready for serving.

2. Heat the oil in a large skillet over medium-high heat. Add the garlic and red pepper flakes, if desired. Sauté for 30 seconds until aromatic. Add the carrots and sauté for 2 to 3 minutes until slightly softened. Add the zucchini, red pepper, and asparagus and cook for 2 minutes. Add the peas and salt and cook until the vegetables are just crisp-tender, about 2 more minutes.

3. Just before the pasta is cooked, reserve 3 tablespoons of the pasta water and add it to the vegetables. Drain the pasta in a colander and add it to the vegetables in the skillet. Add the lemon juice, ½ cup of the Parmesan cheese, and the parsley and toss well.

4. Top each bowl with an extra sprinkle of Parmesan cheese and serve immediately with the remaining cheese on the side.

UDON NOODLE BOWL with PRAWNS

SERVES 6, **VEG***, **V***

Udon are thick wheat noodles greatly enjoyed at noodle houses in Japan; they are served hot in broth with various toppings, or chilled with a dipping sauce and garnishes. Dried udon are widely available in natural-food stores, Asian groceries, and online. Here they appear as sesame noodles with prawns. You might be tempted to eat a huge bowl, but the tahini-based sauce is so rich that you can be perfectly content with a modest portion. Baked, pressed tofu or leftover cooked salmon can substitute for the prawns.

NOODLES

1 (8-ounce) package udon noodles

SAUCE

2 garlic cloves, pressed and allowed to sit for 10 minutes

1 cup tahini

3 tablespoons low-sodium soy sauce

3 tablespoons unseasoned rice vinegar

2 teaspoons lime juice

1 tablespoon minced peeled ginger

¼ teaspoon cayenne pepper

PRAWNS

1 pound cooked prawns

2 tablespoons roughly chopped fresh cilantro leaves

3 scallions, white and light green parts only, thinly sliced

2 tablespoons black sesame seeds

1. In a large pot of salted water, cook the noodles according to the package instructions. Reserve 2 cups of the udon cooking liquid. Drain the noodles in a colander, rinse under cool water, and set aside.

2. Meanwhile, combine all the sauce ingredients with ¼ cup of the noodle cooking water in a medium bowl and stir until smooth.

3. Return the pot to the stove over medium-high heat. Add the cooked noodles, 1 cup of the sauce, and ½ cup of the noodle cooking water, then toss to combine. (Store the extra sauce in an airtight container in the refrigerator for up to 1 week.) If the noodles look too dry, stir in additional noodle water, 1 table-spoon at a time, until the sauce has thinned a bit. Turn off the heat and divide the noodles among 6 serving bowls.

4. Top each portion with the prawns, cilantro, scallions, and black sesame seeds.

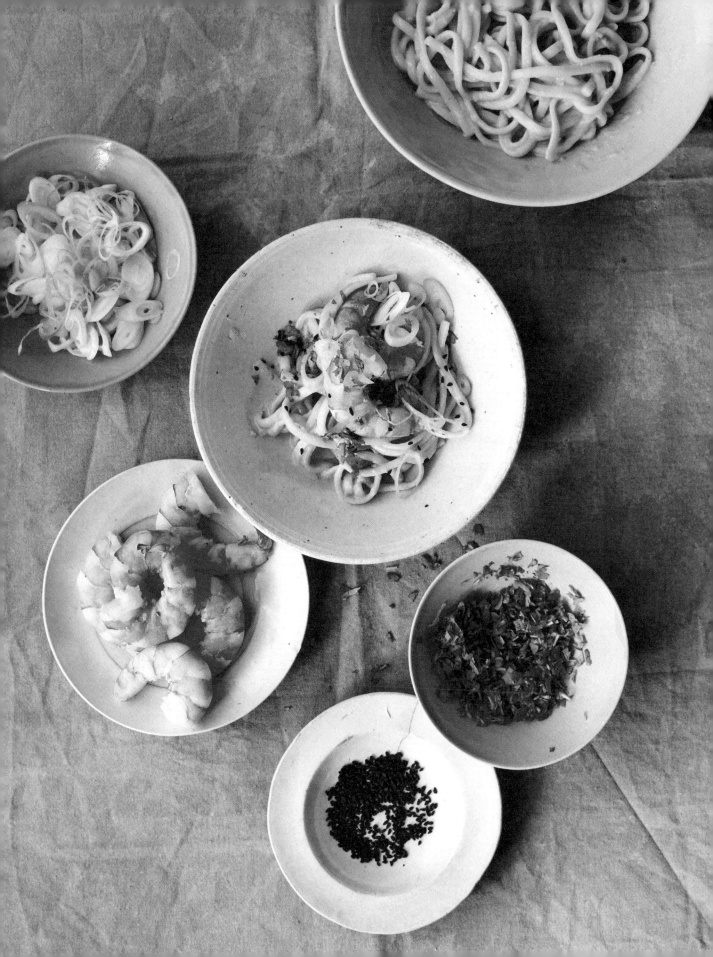

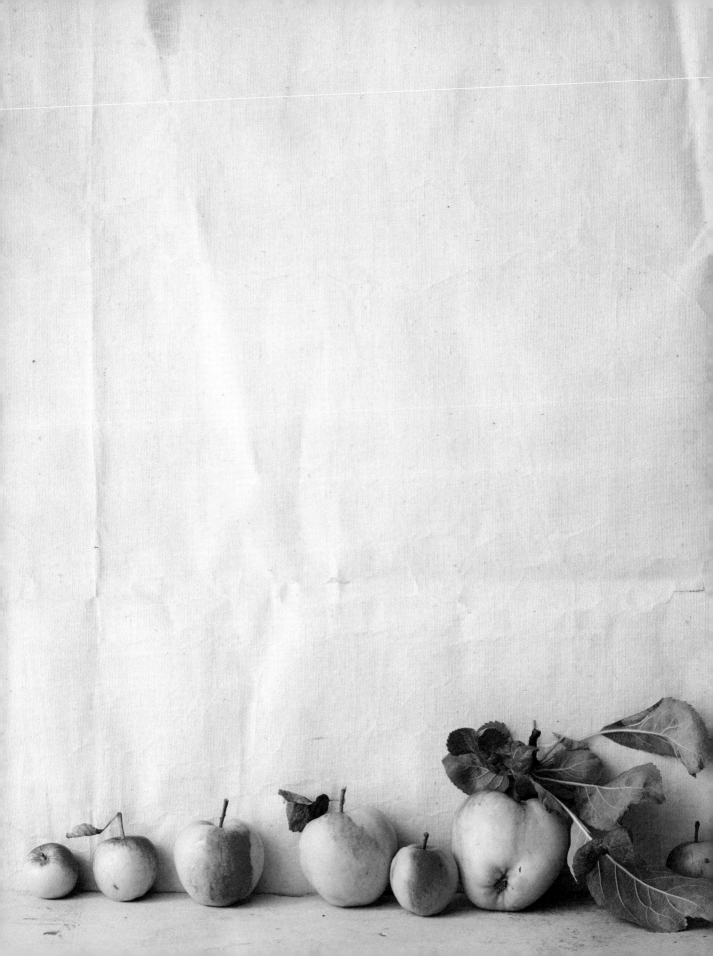

Desserts

I recommend unlearning the habit of ending every meal with a sweet dessert. You can finish a good meal with fruit, cheese, nuts, dark chocolate, or tea rather than pie, cake, or ice cream. As with meats, sugar-laden desserts are occasional items in the Anti-Inflammatory Diet, not everyday ones. I believe the recipes in this section are much better than the decadent indulgences you're likely to be offered in restaurants. Some are versions of familiar sweets made with less sugar and fat; all are easy, delicious, and perfectly fine to enjoy as special treats.

Recipes marked **veg** are vegetarian, those marked **v** are vegan, and those marked **gf** are gluten-free. The symbols **veg***, **v***, and **gf*** indicate recipes that can be modified to be vegetarian, vegan, or gluten-free by substituting or omitting specific ingredients.

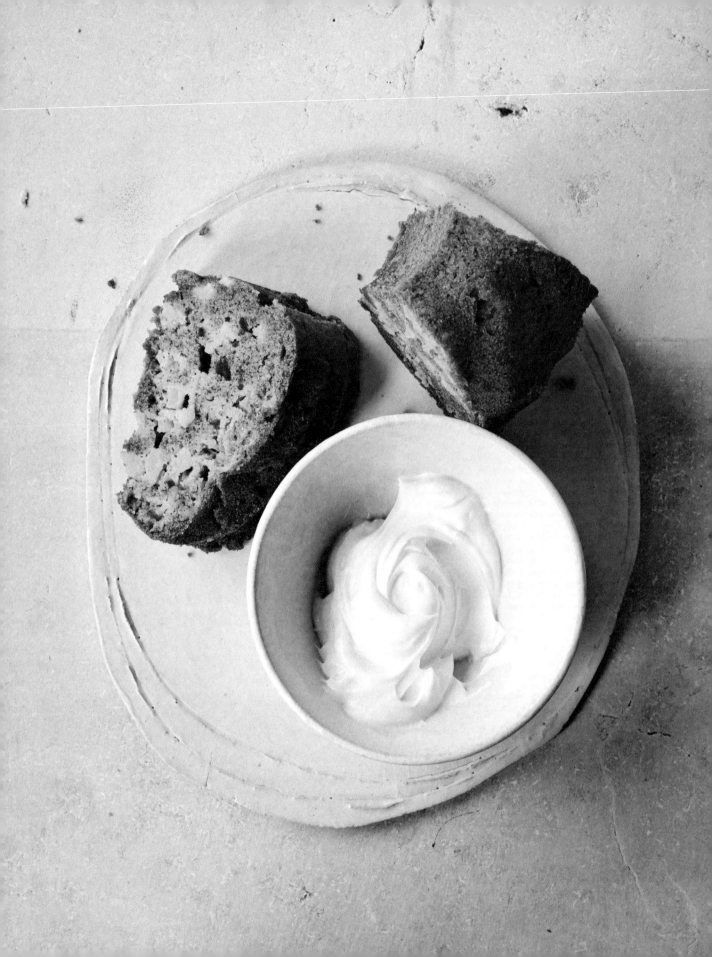

BETTER-THAN-AN-APPLE-A-DAY CAKE

SERVES 16, **VEG**

Olive oil cakes are Italian specialties. Most that I've tried are made with citrus fruit, lemons or oranges. This very moist cake is bursting with fresh apples and fragrant with cinnamon. Because the cake is fairly low in sugar, apples that balance tart with sweet, like Pink Lady, Fuji, or Honey Crisp, are a good choice. Granny Smiths are too tart and don't break down enough in baking. The mix of organic all-purpose flour and teff flour adds a slightly nutty taste. Preparation is quick, but this cake has to bake for an hour, then cool briefly. It is delicious served plain, and fabulous with a scoop of good vanilla ice cream or vanilla yogurt. Any leftover cake can be frozen for up to 3 months.

2 large eggs

¾ cup evaporated cane sugar

¾ cup extra-virgin olive oil (choose one that's fruity, not peppery), plus a little for greasing the pan

1¾ cups all-purpose flour

¼ cup teff flour

1 teaspoon sea salt

1½ teaspoons ground cinnamon

1 teaspoon baking soda

½ teaspoon baking powder

1 teaspoon vanilla extract

¼ cup applesauce

4 apples, peeled, cored, and cut into ¼-inch dice

1. Preheat the oven to 350°F and lightly grease a 10- to 12-cup Bundt pan with a little olive oil.

2. Combine the eggs and sugar in the bowl of an electric mixer. Using the paddle attachment, mix on medium speed for 2 to 3 minutes until pale yellow in color. Add the oil and mix until well incorporated.

3. Whisk or sift together the flours, salt, cinnamon, baking soda, and baking powder. Slowly add the flours to the batter until they're fully incorporated. Add the vanilla, applesauce, and diced apples and mix on low until just combined.

4. Pour the batter into the prepared pan and bake for 55 to 60 minutes or until a toothpick comes out clean. Allow the cake to rest on a cooling rack in the pan for 10 minutes, then invert it onto a rack to cool fully.

APPLE-CRANBERRY FRUIT CRISP

SERVES 8 TO 10, **VEG**

This is a perfect fall dessert. I use Pippin, Pink Lady, or Fuji apples, but these may not be readily available, so a mix of Granny Smith and Fuji is fine. (I like using two different types of apples to get a contrast of tart and sweet.) Almond paste in the topping takes the crisp to another level.

½ cup evaporated cane sugar

4 teaspoons arrowroot powder

¾ teaspoon ground cinnamon

6 to 7 apples, peeled, cored, and cut into ½-inch pieces (about 8 cups)

¼ cup dried cranberries

½ cup (8 tablespoons) unsalted butter

½ cup almond paste

1 cup packed muscovado sugar

½ teaspoon sea salt

½ cup all-purpose flour

½ cup whole-wheat pastry flour

1 cup old-fashioned rolled oats

Vanilla ice cream or frozen yogurt, for serving (optional)

1. Preheat the oven to 350°F.

2. Combine the sugar, arrowroot, and cinnamon in a large bowl. Add the apples and cranberries and toss thoroughly to coat. Divide the fruit mixture among eight 8-ounce ramekins or spread in a 2-quart baking dish.

3. To make the topping, put the butter, almond paste, sugar, and salt in a food processor. Pulse to combine. Add the flours and pulse 2 or 3 times to combine. Transfer to a bowl and fold in the oats. Top the ramekins or baking dish with the topping.

4. Bake for 45 to 50 minutes or until the top is golden, the apples are tender when pierced with a knife, and the juices are bubbling. Serve warm, with vanilla ice cream or frozen yogurt, if desired.

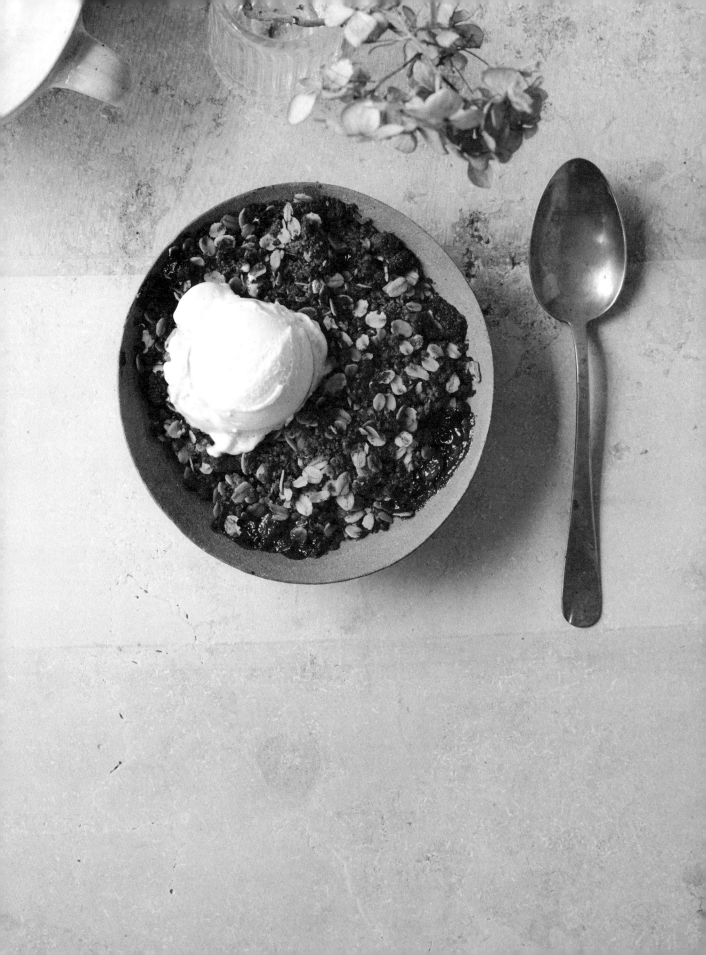

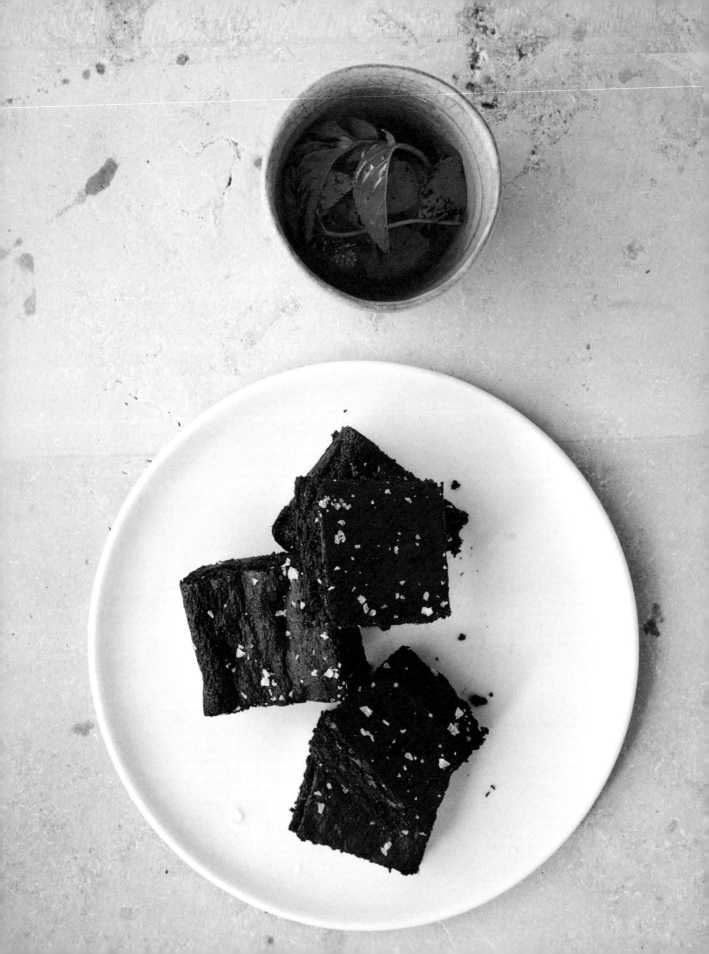

RIDICULOUSLY GOOD
TRIPLE CHOCOLATE BROWNIES

MAKES 16, **VEG**, **GF**

These brownies are really fudgy. They have no gluten and are made with olive oil instead of butter, although you would never know it by tasting them. High-quality chocolate is a must here; use only one with a 68 to 72 percent cacao content. (Note that cacao content is the amount of pure cocoa bean in a chocolate product; the higher the percentage, the more chocolate, which also means more antioxidants and less sugar.) The finishing pinch of fleur de sel takes these brownies over the top.

⅔ cup almond flour

2 tablespoons natural unsweetened cocoa powder

½ teaspoon ground cinnamon

½ teaspoon baking soda

⅛ teaspoon sea salt

8 ounces chopped dark chocolate

⅓ cup extra-virgin olive oil

2 large eggs

⅔ cup evaporated cane sugar

1 teaspoon vanilla extract

2 tablespoons cocoa nibs

Pinch of fleur de sel or fine sea salt

1. Preheat the oven to 350°F and lightly oil an 8-by-8-inch baking pan.

2. Put the almond flour, cocoa powder, cinnamon, baking soda, and salt in a bowl and stir to combine.

3. Put half of the chocolate in a heatproof bowl and set the bowl over a saucepan of simmering water. Heat, stirring often, just until the chocolate is melted and smooth. Remove from the heat and whisk in the olive oil.

4. Crack the eggs into a large bowl and whisk until frothy. Slowly add the sugar, whisking all the while, and continue whisking until the mixture is smooth. Add the vanilla extract, then gradually add the chocolate, whisking vigorously all the while, and continue whisking until smooth and glossy.

5. Add the flour mixture and stir until just combined. Stir in the remaining chocolate and the cocoa nibs. Scrape the mixture into the prepared pan and smooth the top with a spatula.

6. Bake for 15 minutes, then sprinkle with a pinch of fleur de sel. Continue to bake for another 10 minutes or until a toothpick inserted in the center comes out clean. Let cool to room temperature in the pan before cutting. Brownies that don't get eaten right away can be stored in the freezer in a zip-top bag for up to a month.

LEMON and OLIVE OIL CUSTARD

MAKES ABOUT 2 CUPS, SERVES 4, **VEG, GF**

Using olive oil along with a little bit of butter gives this very lemony custard a unique and appealing flavor. Garnish with a little lemon zest and a drizzle of your best extra-virgin olive oil for a lovely finish.

⅓ cup evaporated cane sugar

Zest of 1 lemon, plus more for garnish

½ cup lemon juice

⅛ teaspoon sea salt

4 large eggs, whisked well

2 tablespoons unsalted butter, cut into 2 pieces

2 tablespoons extra-virgin olive oil, plus more for finishing

1. Prepare a double boiler by setting the bottom pot filled with 2 inches of water over medium heat and bring to a simmer. Alternatively, you can set a stainless-steel bowl over a pot of water. The bowl should not be touching the water.

2. In the top pot or stainless-steel bowl, whisk together the sugar, lemon zest, lemon juice, and salt. Whisk in the eggs, then place the pot or bowl over the simmering water and whisk constantly for 5 to 7 minutes, until the mixture thickens and running the whisk through the mixture leaves a trail.

3. Remove from the heat and allow the custard to cool slightly. While still warm, whisk in butter 1 piece at a time and then slowly drizzle in the olive oil. Whisk until the custard is smooth, thick, and silky. Pass the custard through a strainer to catch any solidified egg, pour into a large container, a tart crust (9- or 10-inch), or individual serving cups. Chill for at least an hour in the refrigerator.

4. Before serving, drizzle with olive oil and a few shavings of lemon zest.

CASHEW BRITTLE

SERVES 4, **V**, **GF**

You can think of this treat as a "dessert accessory" that adds a delicate crunch to frozen desserts, like Cashew Scream (page 229) and sorbet, or the Port-Infused Fruit (page 241). It can also take the place of a cookie. The brittle holds up well in an airtight container at room temperature. I can't imagine that you'll have it around for long, but you can freeze it for longer storage.

½ teaspoon grapeseed oil

3 tablespoons grade B maple syrup

2 tablespoons roughly chopped raw cashews

¼ teaspoon ground nutmeg

⅛ teaspoon vanilla extract

⅛ teaspoon sea salt

1. Preheat the oven to 375°F. Line a rimmed baking sheet with parchment paper and spread the oil in a thin even layer.

2. Combine the remaining ingredients in a small bowl. Pour the mixture onto the oiled parchment paper and spread it in an even and thin layer. Bake for about 5 to 7 minutes, staying close to the oven to monitor the baking and avoid burning. The syrup will become bubbly, then after another 2 to 3 minutes, the cashews will take on a golden color and the syrup a deep amber.

3. Remove the brittle from the oven and let it cool to room temperature on the sheet. To make it easier to break, you can pop it in the freezer for about 5 minutes. Break into irregular-size pieces.

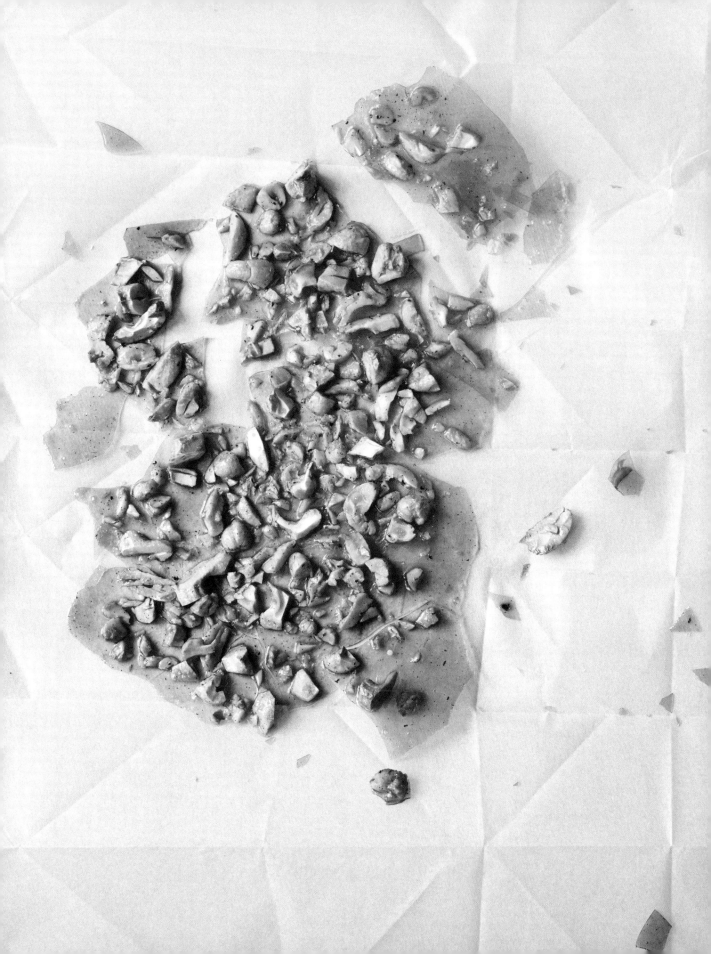

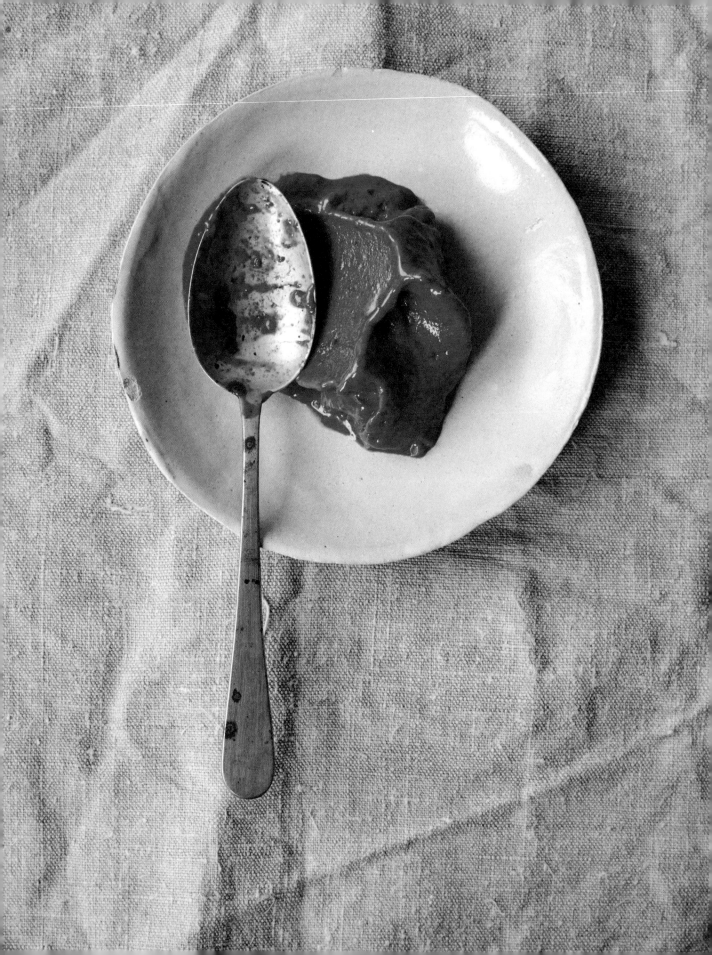

CASHEW SCREAM

SERVES 2, **V, GF**

"I scream, you scream, we all scream for ice cream!" Even though this frozen dessert is vegan, it will still make you scream with delight. The richness and butter-like flavor of Cashew Milk are just right for creating a quick and satisfying frozen treat. Use this recipe as a blueprint—the variations are endless.

1 cup frozen berries

½ cup Cashew Milk (page 275)

1 tablespoon grade B maple syrup

Pinch of sea salt

½ teaspoon vanilla extract

Place the berries in the bowl of a mini food prep or food processor. Pulse the berries about 10 times. Then, add the cashew milk, maple syrup, salt, and vanilla. Blend until smooth. (You can also make this easily with an immersion blender.) Serve immediately.

VARIATIONS: Try 1 cup frozen cherries and 1 tablespoon finely chopped dark chocolate, or 1 cup frozen peaches and ½ teaspoon ground ginger.

COCONUT-LEMON BARS

SERVES 16, **VEG**

This is a healthier riff on the classic lemon bar. Instead of butter, it uses olive oil, ground hazelnuts, and coconut to create a satisfying shortbread crust. The lemon-curd custard is made with much less sugar than usual. A very satisfying treat.

CRUST

½ cup rolled oats

3 tablespoons hazelnuts

1 tablespoon plus 1 teaspoon all-purpose flour

¼ teaspoon sea salt

6 tablespoons shredded unsweetened coconut

4½ tablespoons grade B maple syrup

1½ tablespoons extra-virgin olive oil

FILLING

1 tablespoon plus 1 teaspoon grated lemon zest

¾ cup lemon juice

¾ cup grade B maple syrup

4 large eggs

6 tablespoons all-purpose flour, sifted

⅛ teaspoon sea salt

2 tablespoons toasted coconut (page 274)

1. Preheat the oven to 375°F. Lightly oil an 8-by-8-inch square baking pan.

2. Pulse the oats, hazelnuts, flour, and salt together in a food processor until the ingredients resemble a coarse meal. Add the coconut, maple syrup, and oil and pulse until all the ingredients are evenly moist but still crumbly-looking.

3. Transfer the mixture to the pan and press it evenly and firmly into the bottom with wet fingers to prevent it from sticking to you. Bake for 15 to 16 minutes or until set. Remove from the oven and let cool, but keep the oven on.

4. With a stand or a hand mixer, beat the filling ingredients except the toasted coconut until fluffy and well combined. Pour the filling over the crust and bake for 15 minutes or until set.

5. Let cool completely and top with toasted coconut. Cut into 16 squares. These store well in the freezer. Wrap squares individually in wax paper or parchment, seal in a zip-top bag, and freeze for up to a month.

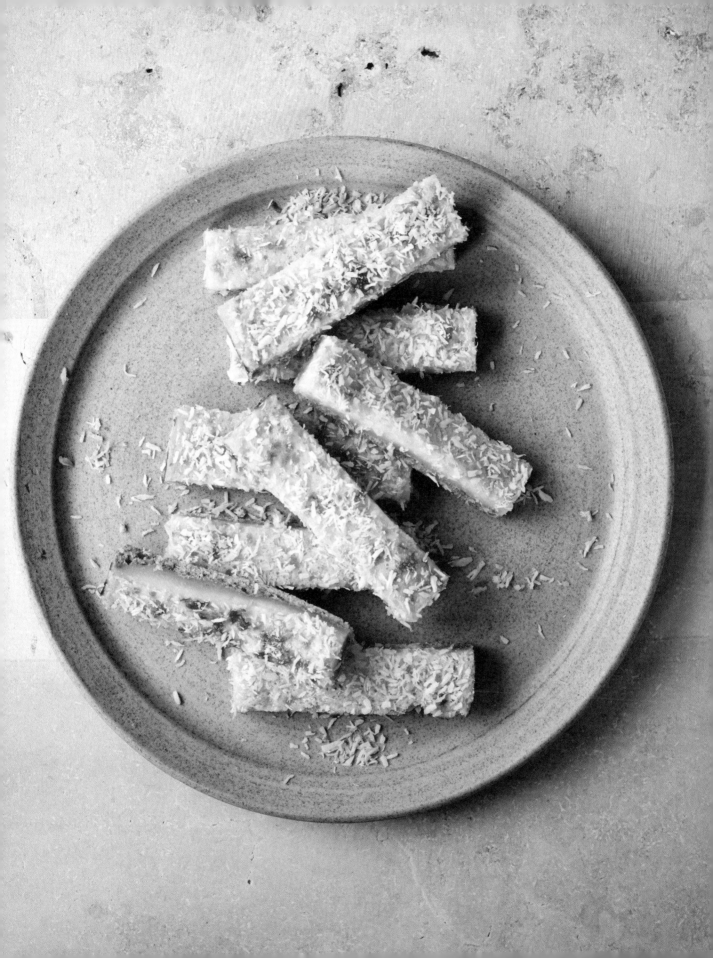

DARK CHOCOLATE DATE
and NUT TRUFFLES

MAKES 20 TRUFFLES, **V, GF**

This recipe is a slam-dunk no matter what your cooking-skill level. Even nonbakers will have success. I first tasted these creations of Rebecca Katz in 2011 in San Francisco at the Arizona Center for Integrative Medicine's Nutrition and Health Conference. I asked Rebecca for the recipe, and since then, it's become one of my go-tos. It's great for company since it makes 20 truffles.

¼ cup finely diced dried apricots or dried cranberries

2 ounces dark chocolate (64 to 72 percent cacao content), finely chopped

⅓ cup plus 2 tablespoons raw almonds

1 cup pitted and halved Medjool dates

1½ teaspoons grated orange zest or ½ teaspoon orange oil (not extract)

⅛ teaspoon sea salt

½ cup unsweetened shredded coconut

1. Soak the apricots or cranberries in cold water for 5 minutes.

2. Place the chopped chocolate in a small bowl and stir in 2 tablespoons of boiling water. Let stand for 30 seconds. Using a small whisk, stir until the chocolate is completely melted and glossy.

3. Coarsely grind the almonds in a food processor, then add the dates, orange zest or oil, salt, and the chocolate and process until smooth, about 1 minute. Transfer to a bowl; drain the apricots or cranberries well and stir them into the chocolate mixture. Cover and chill for approximately 2 hours, until firm.

4. Scatter the coconut on a large plate. Scoop up 1 tablespoon of the chocolate mixture and roll it into a smooth ball between your palms, then roll it in the coconut to coat. Repeat with the remaining mixture, then place the truffles in an airtight container and chill thoroughly before serving. They will keep in the refrigerator for up to 3 days.

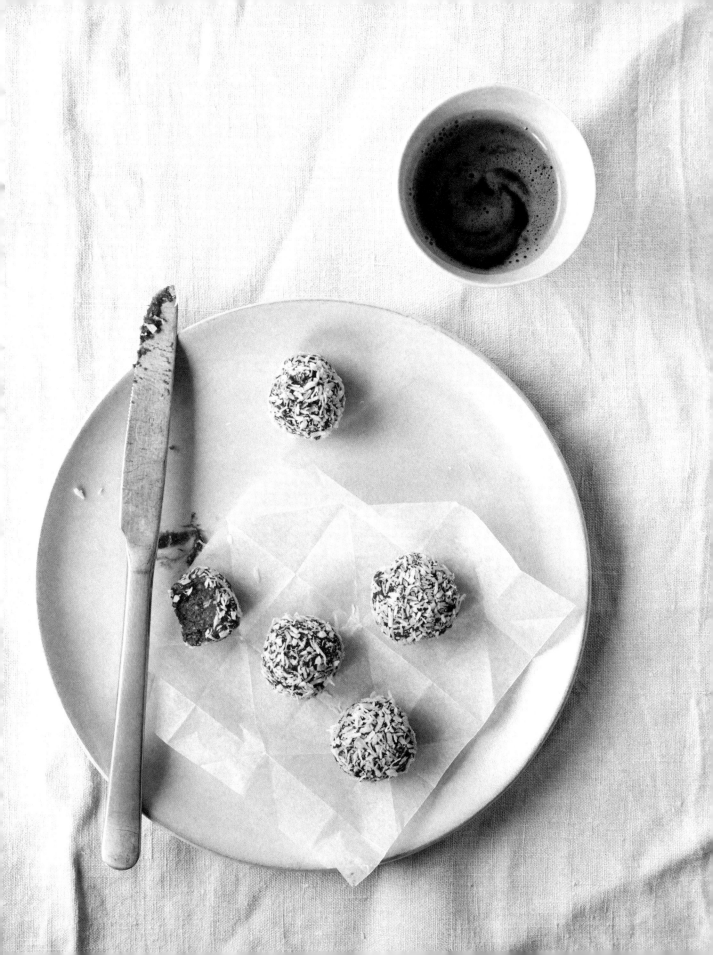

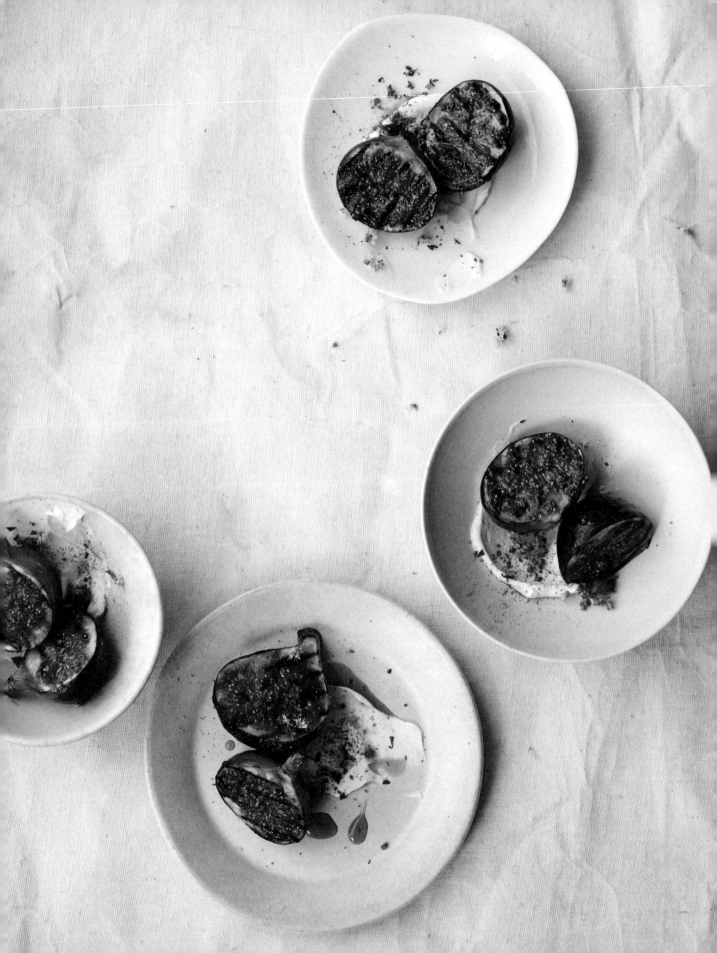

GRILLED FIGS with VANILLA-SCENTED MASCARPONE

SERVES 4, **VEG, GF**

When fresh figs are available, try this wonderful dessert that's both fast and elegant. With just a quick moment on the grill, the figs become jammy. The figs, maple, cinnamon, nutmeg, and vanilla-scented mascarpone are a match made in heaven. (You could substitute Greek yogurt or ricotta for the mascarpone.) You can also serve this at breakfast.

1 tablespoon extra-virgin olive oil

8 ripe but firm fresh figs, halved

1 tablespoon grade B maple syrup

1 teaspoon ground cinnamon

½ cup mascarpone cheese

½ teaspoon vanilla extract

Sprinkle of ground nutmeg

Fresh spearmint leaves, sliced

1. Heat a grill or grill pan over medium-high heat. Rub the olive oil onto the cut sides of the figs. Place on the grill, flat-side down, for about 2 to 3 minutes or until grill marks appear. Turn the figs over using tongs or a spatula and grill for another 2 to 3 minutes on the other side.

2. Remove the figs to a platter, then brush each fig on the cut side with maple syrup and sprinkle with cinnamon.

3. Meanwhile, mix together the mascarpone and vanilla extract in a small bowl. Top each fig with a dollop of the cheese mixture and a shaving of nutmeg. Garnish the platter with spearmint and serve immediately.

NORI'S ORANGE-COCONUT MACAROONS

MAKES 12 COOKIES, **VEG, GF**

My longtime friend and master gardener from Cortes Island, British Columbia, Nori Fletcher makes these very easy, low-fat treats. (They are also gluten-free.) They should be a bit moist and chewy, subtly flavored with the orange zest and liqueur. If you're a chocolate lover, by all means add ¼ cup of mini–chocolate chips to the batter.

2 egg whites

½ cup evaporated cane sugar

2 cups desiccated unsweetened coconut

Zest of 1 orange

1 tablespoon Grand Marnier liqueur

1 teaspoon vanilla extract

⅛ teaspoon sea salt

1. Preheat the oven to 350°F. Line a baking sheet with parchment paper.

2. Whisk together the egg whites and sugar until the sugar is mostly dissolved. Add the remaining ingredients and mix well.

3. Pack 2 tablespoons of dough into a scoop, then gently place the dough ball onto the baking sheet; the balls should be about 2 inches apart. (The dough will be a bit crumbly and may fall apart. Press back into shape.)

4. Bake for 18 minutes or until lightly browned. Allow to cool for about 10 minutes before removing to a cooling rack. Store in an airtight container for up to 5 days or freeze for up to 2 months.

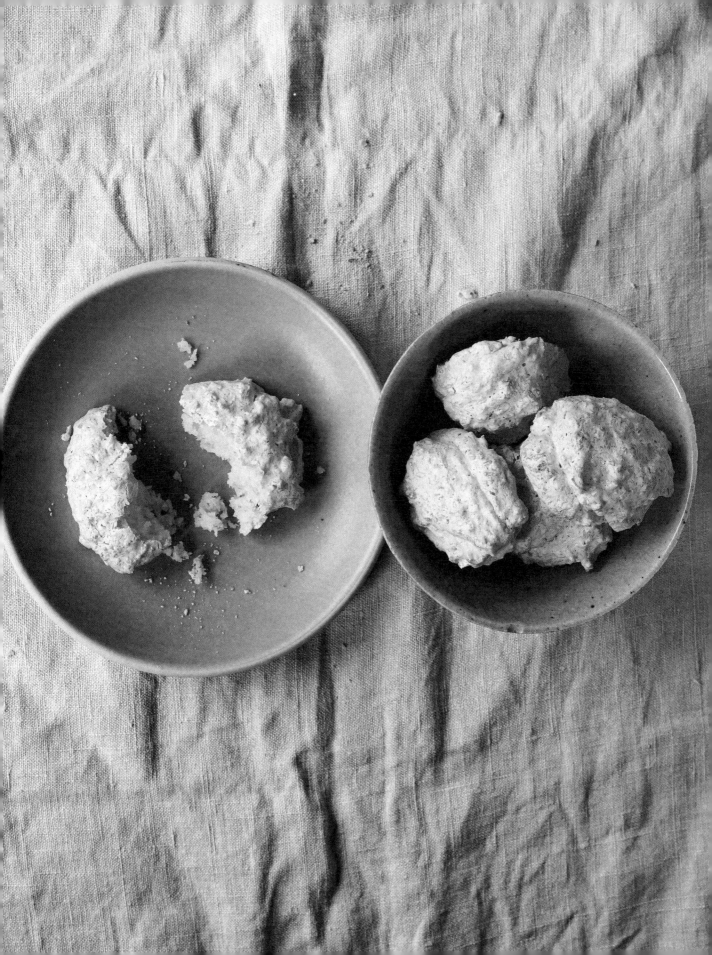

GINGER-PEACH SORBET

MAKES 1 QUART, SERVES 4 TO 6, **V, GF**

Peaches and ginger are a winning combination. (Nectarines or plums would work here too.) Really ripe peaches peel easily and are so sweet that you need less sugar than you'd expect to turn them into a sorbet. I like going to farmers' markets during stone-fruit season to pick out the overripe peaches that farmers are willing to almost give away.

2 teaspoons lemon juice

1 tablespoon grated peeled ginger

¼ cup evaporated cane sugar

Pinch of sea salt

6 ripe peaches (about 3 pounds),
pitted, peeled, and coarsely chopped

1. Chill the ice cream machine canister in the freezer according to manufacturer's directions.

2. In a pot over medium-high heat, add 1 cup of water, the lemon juice, ginger, sugar, and salt and whisk until the sugar has dissolved. Add the peaches and cook until they have softened, about 5 minutes.

3. Pour the fruit and 1 more cup of water into a blender and puree until silky-smooth. Refrigerate the puree until chilled, about 1 to 2 hours; it must be cold before going into the ice cream machine. Then freeze according to your ice cream maker's directions.

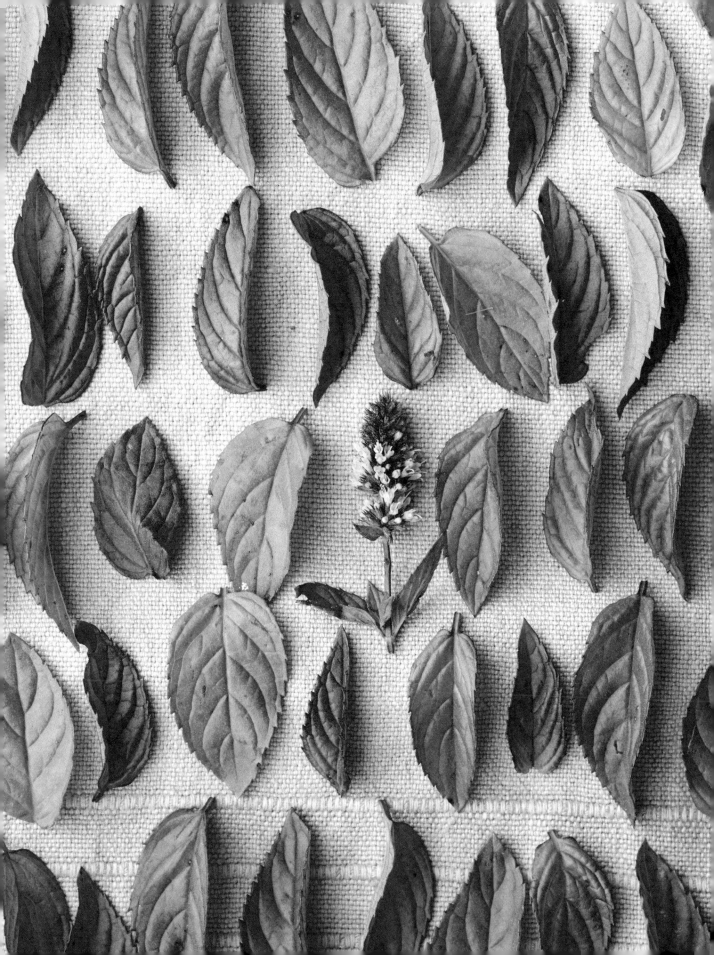

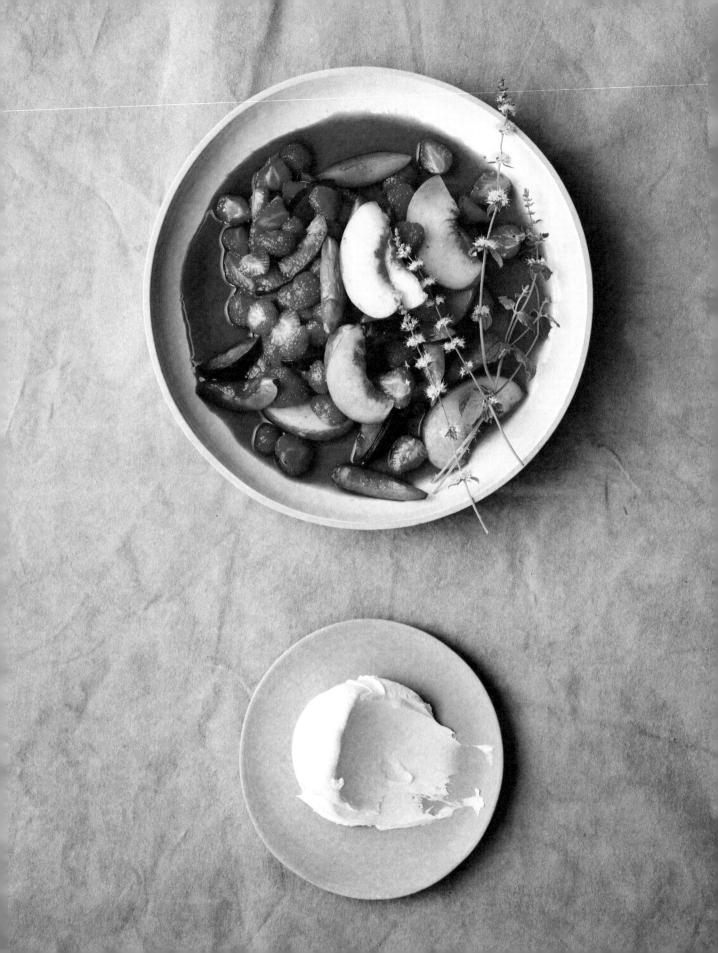

PORT-INFUSED FRUIT
with MASCARPONE CHEESE

SERVES 8, **VEG, GF**

Maceration is the process of soaking fruit in a flavorful liquid. The fruit absorbs some of the liquid, which softens it and enhances its taste. Sweet port wine is ideal for this. Adding mascarpone, a soft Italian cheese made from cream and often used in desserts, makes this richer and more substantial.

1 pint strawberries, sliced

4 plums, pitted and sliced

2 peaches, pitted and sliced

2 tablespoons evaporated cane sugar

3 tablespoons tawny port wine

8 ounces mascarpone cheese, at room temperature

Thinly sliced fresh spearmint leaves (optional)

1. Place the fruit in a large glass mixing bowl. Toss it with the sugar and port. Let the fruit macerate for 20 minutes at room temperature, occasionally tossing it with a spoon.

2. Meanwhile, divide the mascarpone among 8 bowls. Top each portion with about ½ cup of fruit and drizzle over a scant tablespoon of the liquid from the bottom of the bowl. Garnish with fresh spearmint if desired and serve right away.

NOTE: You can substitute 2 additional cups of strawberries for the plums and peaches.

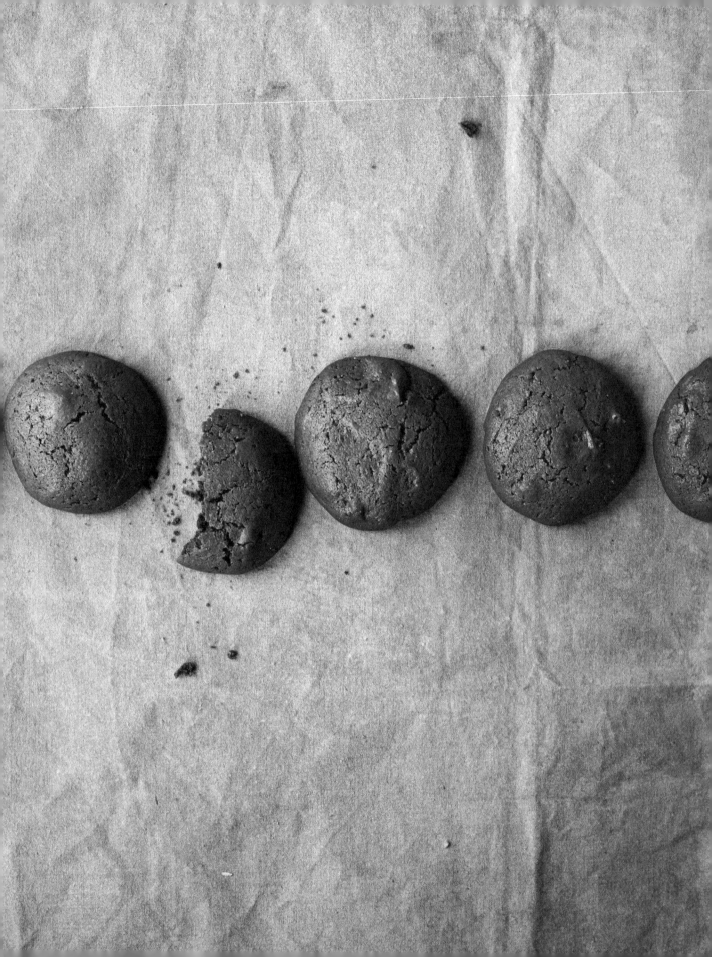

GINGER MOLASSES COOKIES

MAKES ABOUT 24 (2-INCH) COOKIES, **VEG**

This recipe is an homage to the healing and warming spice ginger, since it's utilized three different ways. Ginger in all forms is a powerful natural anti-inflammatory agent. The molasses makes for a really earthy cookie.

2¼ cups spelt or all-purpose flour

½ teaspoon baking soda

½ teaspoon sea salt

½ cup evaporated cane sugar

½ cup blackstrap molasses

½ cup extra-virgin olive oil

1 teaspoon ground ginger

¾ teaspoon ground cinnamon

¼ teaspoon ground cloves

¼ teaspoon ground nutmeg

1 teaspoon grated peeled ginger

1 egg

½ cup chopped candied (crystallized) ginger

1. Preheat the oven to 350°F and line two baking sheets with parchment or silicone mats.

2. Whisk or sift together the flour, baking soda, and salt and set aside.

3. In the mixing bowl of a stand mixer fitted with the paddle attachment, combine the sugar, molasses, oil, ground spices, and grated ginger on medium-low. Beat until the mixture has a glossy appearance, about 3 minutes. Add the egg and beat until well combined. Add in the dry ingredients, mix until just combined, then fold in the candied ginger. The dough will be thick and sticky.

4. Lightly oil a tablespoon, then drop spoonfuls of the dough spaced 2 inches apart onto the baking sheets. You should be able to fit 12 cookies per sheet.

5. Bake for about 13 minutes. The cookies will still feel soft, but the tops will appear dry and begin to crack. Allow to cool for about 5 minutes, then use a spatula to remove to a cooling rack.

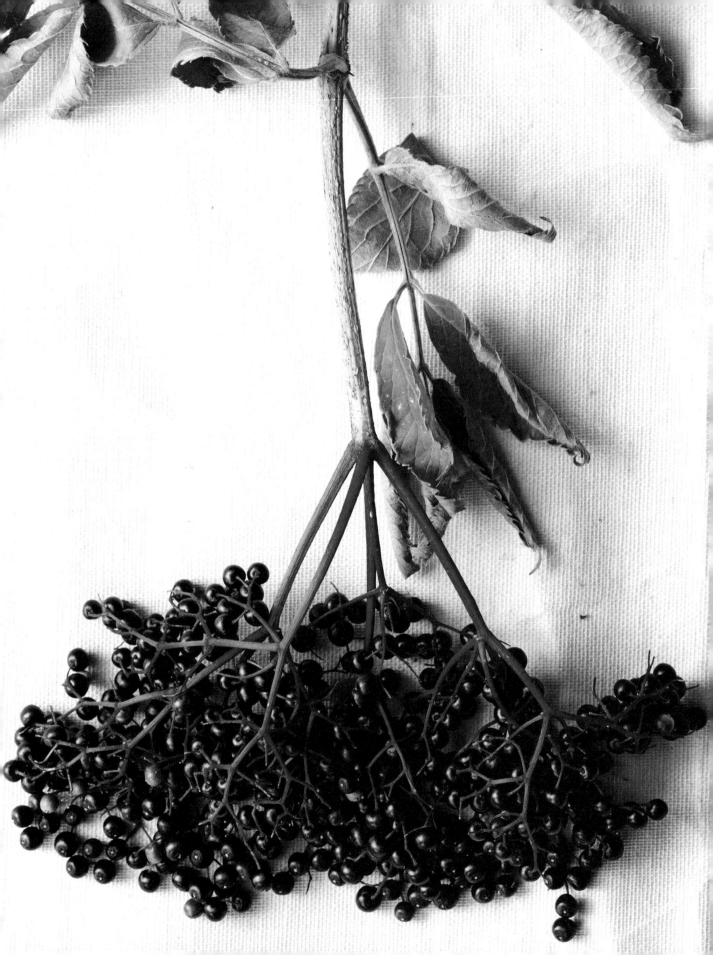

Drinks

The greatest contributor to the obesity epidemic in our population, especially in our kids, is probably sweetened drinks—not just soda but also fruit juice, sweetened coffee and tea, and energy drinks. I got out of the habit of drinking sweet liquids long ago. My favorite drink now is water—if it's pure. I also love sparkling water, plain or with a bit of lemon or lime, and, on occasion, unsweetened iced tea. If I want alcohol, I prefer red wine and cold sake. I've put some creative drink recipes in this section, including a few cocktails and some colorful combinations of fruit and vegetable juices, most with little or no added sweeteners. Try some with breakfast (not the cocktails); use others with starters when guests arrive.

Recipes marked **veg** are vegetarian, those marked **v** are vegan, and those marked **gf** are gluten-free. The symbols **veg***, **v***, and **gf*** indicate recipes that can be modified to be vegetarian, vegan, or gluten-free by substituting or omitting specific ingredients.

BLACK SESAME SMOOTHIE

SERVES 2, **VEG, GF**

Rich and satisfying, this smoothie needs little added sweetener if the bananas are very ripe (with thin, heavily spotted skins and no green ends). Ground black sesame seeds enhance the appearance, texture, and taste of the drink. It is good with breakfast.

¼ cup black sesame seeds

2 large, very ripe bananas

2½ cups soymilk or cashew milk

¼ cup kefir

1 teaspoon grade B maple syrup

4 to 6 ice cubes

1. In a dry skillet, lightly toast the sesame seeds over medium heat until fragrant. Let them cool for a minute, then grind as fine as possible in an electric spice grinder.

2. Place all the ingredients in a blender and blend until smooth, adding more soymilk or cashew milk by the tablespoon until you reach a nice creamy consistency.

3. Pour into 2 chilled glasses and serve.

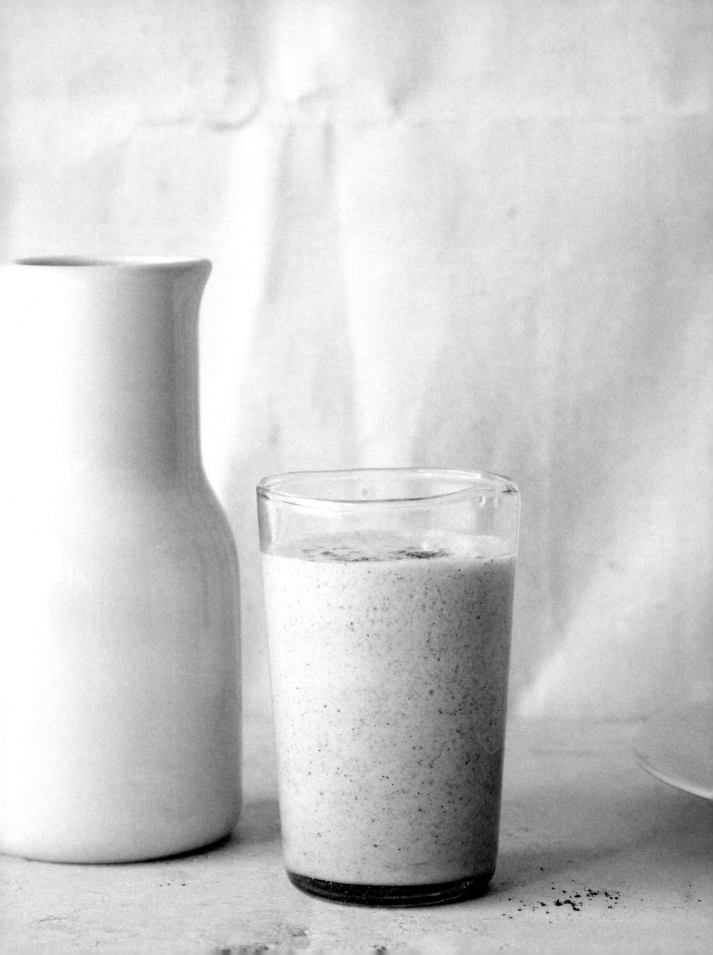

CUCUMBER CRANBERRY COOLER

SERVES 4, **V, GF**

Cucumber juice is so refreshing, and here it smooths out the tartness of the cranberry. A little maple syrup is just right.

1 cucumber, peeled, seeded, and diced

12 ounces unsweetened cranberry juice

8 ounces freshly squeezed orange juice

1 tablespoon grade B maple syrup or Maple Simple Syrup (page 275)

4 orange slices (optional)

1. Put the cucumber and 2 tablespoons of water in a blender and puree. Strain the puree through a fine-mesh sieve into a pitcher. You should have close to 1 cup of cucumber juice.

2. In a pitcher, mix together the cucumber juice, ¾ cup of water, the cranberry juice, orange juice, and maple syrup.

3. Pour over ice in 4 tall glasses and garnish each with an orange slice.

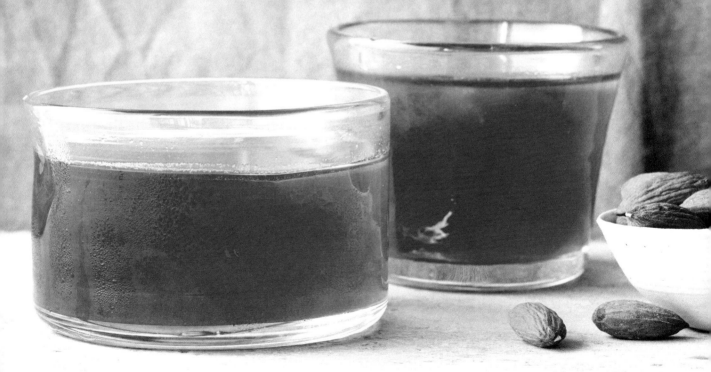

GINGER LIME FIZZ
with FROZEN GRAPES

SERVES 1, **V, GF**

This bubbly delight is as bright and fresh as it is beautiful. (The lime is in the syrup.)
Enjoy it on a hot afternoon!

¼ cup **Ginger-Spearmint Syrup**
(page 277)

Frozen red seedless grapes

6 ounces sparkling water

1 sprig spearmint

Add the Ginger-Spearmint Syrup to a glass with a few frozen grapes, then fill
the glass with sparkling water and garnish with a sprig of spearmint.

GINGERY MATCHA COOLER

SERVES 2, V, GF

Matcha, the bright green powdered tea used in the Japanese tea ceremony, makes a refreshing cold drink. It's available online (from breakawaymatcha.com, matchaand more.com, japanesegreenteaonline.com, inpursuitoftea.com, and other sites). The powder should be sieved before it's mixed with hot water to prevent it from clumping. Store opened *matcha* in the freezer.

2 teaspoons *matcha* powder, rubbed through a fine sieve

1 teaspoon finely grated peeled ginger

2 teaspoons lemon juice

2 teaspoons Maple Simple Syrup (page 275)

8 ice cubes, plus more for serving

2 sprigs spearmint

1. Whisk *matcha* powder and ¼ cup of hot water until the powder is well combined and the color is uniform.

2. Place the *matcha* mixture, ¾ cup of cold water, and the remaining ingredients except the sprigs of spearmint into a blender and puree until smooth. (Or use an immersion blender.)

3. Pour into 2 glasses with ice and garnish each with a sprig of spearmint.

ENERGIZING GREEN TONIC

SERVES 2, V, **GF**

A very simple, refreshing beverage packed with nutritional goodies and a great pick-me-up—a hybrid of a juice and a smoothie. The lemon and apple offset the earthiness of raw spinach. Add more liquid to achieve the consistency you like. If you want this drink a little sweeter, add another half an apple. Try it with breakfast.

1 small cucumber, peeled and cut into chunks

1 stalk celery, cut into chunks

1 green apple, peeled, cored, and cut into chunks

1 cup loosely packed baby spinach

4 romaine lettuce leaves, torn into pieces

1 tablespoon lemon juice

1 teaspoon finely chopped peeled ginger

Pinch of sea salt

1. Put the ingredients and 2 cups of water into a blender and puree on high speed for 1 to 2 minutes, until smooth.

2. Strain through a fine-mesh sieve and serve chilled or over ice.

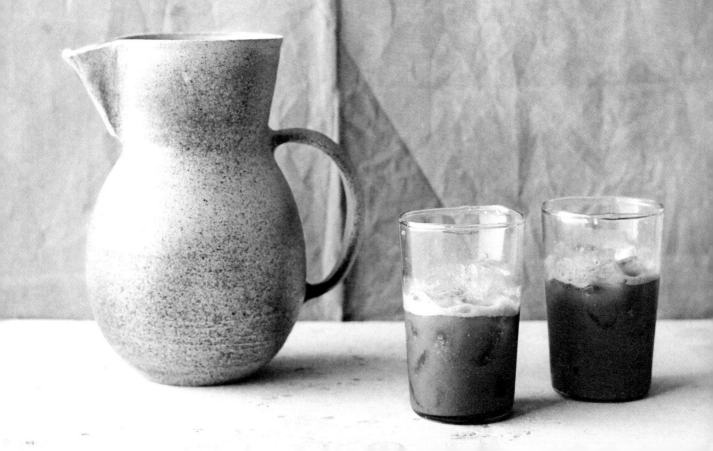

GREEN TEA–BLUEBERRY INFUSION

SERVES 1, **V, GF**

This is a drink to clear any cobwebs from your head. The health benefits of green tea and the antioxidants it contains are well documented; lemon juice increases the antioxidants' bioavailability. Blueberries are rich in protective anthocyanin pigments. No sugar needed. This is good with breakfast.

1 green tea bag

½ cup fresh or frozen blueberries

2 teaspoons lemon juice

1 lemon slice

Put the tea bag in 1 cup of boiling water and let it steep for 5 minutes. Remove the tea bag, then pour the tea, blueberries, and lemon juice into a blender and blend for less than a minute. Strain into a tall glass. Add ice and garnish with a slice of lemon.

BOURBON MANHATTAN

SERVES 1, **V, GF**

Like the sidecar, the Manhattan is one of America's historic cocktails, with literary references going back at least a hundred years. The key ingredients are whiskey, sweet vermouth, bitters, and a maraschino cherry. The drink can be served up in a martini glass or on the rocks in a lowball glass. Maker's Mark Bourbon, a reasonably priced, readily available whiskey, works well here. You can also experiment with rye whiskey (Bulleit rye, for example) to add a slightly spicy complexity to the cocktail. Maraschino cherries that are not packed in high-fructose syrup and dyed fluorescent red are available from Whole Foods Markets, Trader Joe's, natural-food stores, and online. There are numerous bitters products on the market, from common Angostura bitters that you can find in most grocery stores to artisanal products like Fee Brothers Whiskey Barrel-Aged Bitters, available from feebrothers.com.

1½ ounces bourbon

1 ounce sweet vermouth

1 or 2 dashes of bitters

1 maraschino cherry

Place all the ingredients except the cherry in a cocktail shaker with lots of ice. Shake for about 10 seconds and strain into a martini glass or rocks glass with fresh ice. Some prefer this cocktail stirred rather than shaken; if so, follow the same steps but stir the ingredients in your shaker before straining into the glass. Drop in the cherry and enjoy.

VARIATION: For a slightly less sweet cocktail, try the perfect Manhattan. Instead of using all sweet vermouth, substitute ½ ounce sweet vermouth and ½ ounce dry (white) vermouth.

CHEEKY DEVIL

SERVES 1, **V, GF**

This super-easy-to-make cocktail accentuates the aromatic sweetness of St. Germain. Grenadine, a sweet syrup made from red currants and pomegranate juice, is often associated with the fluorescent-red high-fructose-corn-syrup concoctions found on most supermarket shelves. Stay away from those products and instead look for artisanal versions that use only pomegranate juice, cane sugar, and perhaps a bit of lemon juice. Grenadine from Skylake Ranch, a family orchard in Northern California, is excellent; it can be ordered online at skylakeranch.com/products/pomegranate-grenadine. To get the clearest, most beautiful color, store the bottle vertically in your refrigerator and pour carefully to keep the sediment on the bottom. You'll enjoy this drink year-round but especially in the summer.

1½ ounces gin

1 ounce St. Germain elderflower liqueur

½ ounce lime juice

1 teaspoon artisanal grenadine

1 lime slice

Put all the ingredients except the grenadine and lime slice into a cocktail shaker filled with enough ice to cover the liquid. Shake well. Strain out the ice and pour into a chilled glass. Carefully pour in the grenadine. Garnish with the lime slice.

CHEEKY BUBBLE

SERVES 1, **V, GF**

Here's a very easy way to add some interest to Prosecco or moderately priced champagne. St. Germain is a liqueur made from elderflower blossoms that are handpicked, gathered in sacks, and then quaintly taken by bicycle down the French hillside. It adds sweetness to the sparkling wine: experiment with the amount you add.

4 to 6 ounces Prosecco or champagne
¼ to ½ ounce St. Germain elderflower liqueur
1 lemon twist

Pour the well-chilled sparkling wine into a glass.
Add the St. Germain. Drop in the lemon twist.

Cheeky Devil

Cheeky Bubble

FRESH GINGER LIME DROP

SERVES 1, **V, GF**

This cocktail is a "must" for fresh ginger lovers. The key is to muddle the ginger very well in order to loosen it and release its flavor. If you don't have a cocktail muddler, use the handle end of a wooden spoon.

½ ounce orange liqueur, preferably Cointreau or Grand Marnier

¾ ounce artisanal grenadine

2 to 3 thin slices peeled ginger

1½ ounces vodka

1 ounce lime juice

1 thin lime slice

1. Chill a martini glass in the freezer.

2. Pour the orange liqueur and grenadine into the cocktail shaker. Add the ginger slices and muddle them well. Add the vodka, lime juice, and ice and shake vigorously for about 10 seconds. Strain all the ingredients into your cocktail glass and garnish with the lime slice.

KIR DAISY

"Daisy" is the English translation of *margarita*, and this cocktail takes the drink in a whole new direction. Except for the tequila, all the ingredients are different from those in a traditional margarita. The Kir Daisy uses *amaro*, a bittersweet Italian herbal liqueur.

2 ounces 100 percent agave tequila

¾ ounce lemon juice

½ ounce dry (white) vermouth

½ ounce amaro

Place all the ingredients in a cocktail shaker with lots of ice. Shake for about 10 seconds and strain into a martini glass.

CORTES ISLAND CAESAR

SERVES 1, **GF**

The Canadian national drink, the Caesar, was invented in 1969. Immensely popular with Canadians, it is largely unknown to Americans. Essentially, it's a highly spiced and inventively garnished Bloody Mary made with Clamato instead of tomato juice. Clamato is a flavored blend of clam and tomato juices; sadly, it is loaded with high-fructose corn syrup and contains both MSG and artificial red coloring. You can make a healthier Caesar using tomato juice and bottled clam juice (available in most supermarkets). On Cortes Island, British Columbia, we put enough vegetables in the glass to make this an almost-salad as well as a most enjoyable summer drink.

4 ounces tomato juice

1½ ounces vodka

2 teaspoons Prepared Fresh Horseradish (page 268)

1 teaspoon clam juice

2 dashes Worcestershire sauce

Dash of hot sauce

Lime wedge

2 green pitted olives (optional)

2 cocktail onions (optional)

Celery stalk

Cucumber wedge

Trimmed scallion

1. Fill a tall highball glass with ice.

2. Add the tomato juice, vodka, horseradish, clam juice, Worcestershire sauce, and hot sauce and stir well. Squeeze the lime wedge in and drop it into the glass with the olives and onions.

3. Garnish with the celery stalk, cucumber wedge, and scallion.

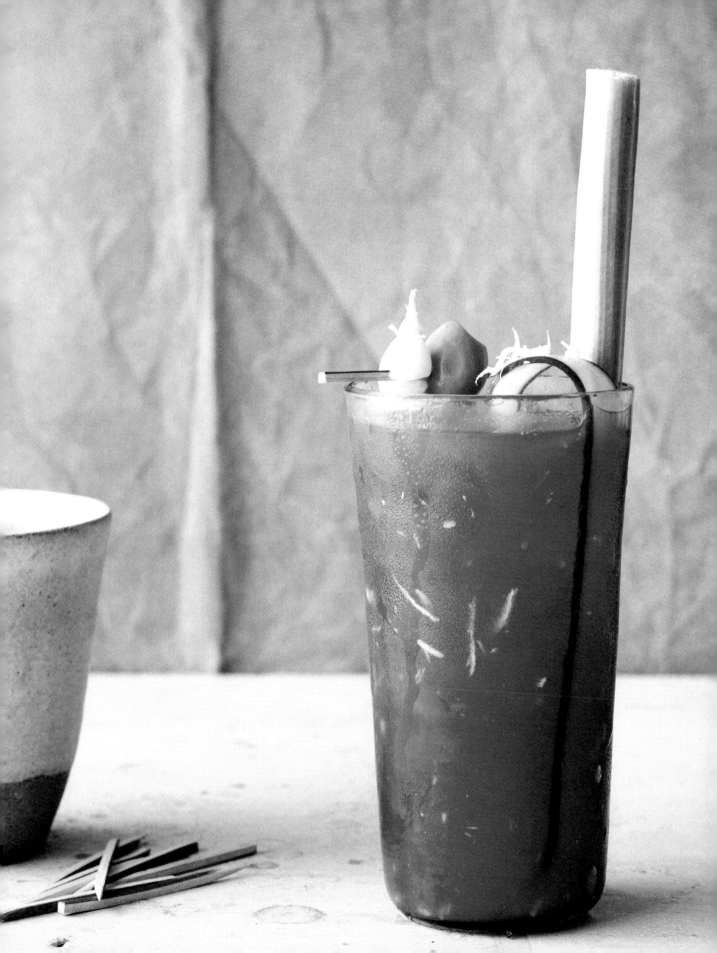

MARGARITAS

SERVES 1, **V**, **GF**

Following are two margarita recipes I think you'll love. They both use only simple, basic ingredients that allow the unique taste of the tequila to come through. (Use only tequila that is clearly marked *100 percent agave*.) Initially, these may seem strong, since they're not diluted with mixers or extra water, but with a little experimentation with the proportions of sweet and sour, you'll be able to create a cocktail that is perfectly balanced and far better than most bar offerings.

BASIC MARGARITA

1½ ounces 100 percent agave tequila

1 ounce lime juice

½ ounce orange liqueur, such as Grand Marnier or Cointreau

½ ounce Maple Simple Syrup (page 275)

1 lime slice

Sea salt (optional)

Place all the ingredients except the lime slice and salt in a cocktail shaker with lots of ice. Shake for about 10 seconds and strain into a rocks glass containing fresh ice. You can also use a margarita glass with a salted rim: run a lime segment around the rim and dip rim lightly into a plate with a thin layer of salt. Garnish with the lime slice.

POMEGRANATE MARGARITA

1½ ounces 100 percent agave tequila

1 ounce lime juice

1 ounce artisanal grenadine

½ ounce pure pomegranate juice

1 lime slice

Place the first three ingredients in a cocktail shaker with lots of ice. Shake for about 10 seconds and strain into a rocks glass containing fresh ice. Drizzle the pure pomegranate juice on top and garnish with the lime slice.

VERMONT BLUEGRASS

SERVES 1, **V, GF**

Here is another bourbon drink that you can enjoy as the evenings begin to get chilly with the approach of fall.

1½ ounces bourbon

½ tablespoon Maple Cinnamon Simple Syrup (page 276)

½ tablespoon lemon juice

½ tablespoon Cointreau

Cinnamon stick

Place the first four ingredients in a cocktail shaker with ice. Shake gently for about 10 seconds and pour into a cocktail glass. Add the cinnamon stick and serve.

MEYER SIDECAR

SERVES 1, **V, GF**

This is a slight variation on an all-time classic cocktail that first appeared in print in 1907 and has endured ever since. I suggest using Rémy Martin VSOP Cognac, generally available for under forty dollars; one of the better brandies will also do. You can substitute triple sec for Cointreau, but this will reduce the quality of the finished drink.

1½ ounces cognac

1 ounce Meyer lemon juice (see Note)

1 ounce Cointreau

¼ orange slice

Chill a martini glass in the freezer. Put all the ingredients except the orange slice into a cocktail shaker and fill with ice. Shake vigorously for at least 15 seconds but no more than 20. Strain the golden concoction into the glass and garnish with a quarter of an orange slice.

VARIATION: For a delicious alternative, you can make a Caribbean sidecar. Follow the recipe above but substitute Ten Cane Rum for the cognac.

NOTE: If you don't have Meyer lemons, mix the juice of a fresh orange with the juice of a lemon.

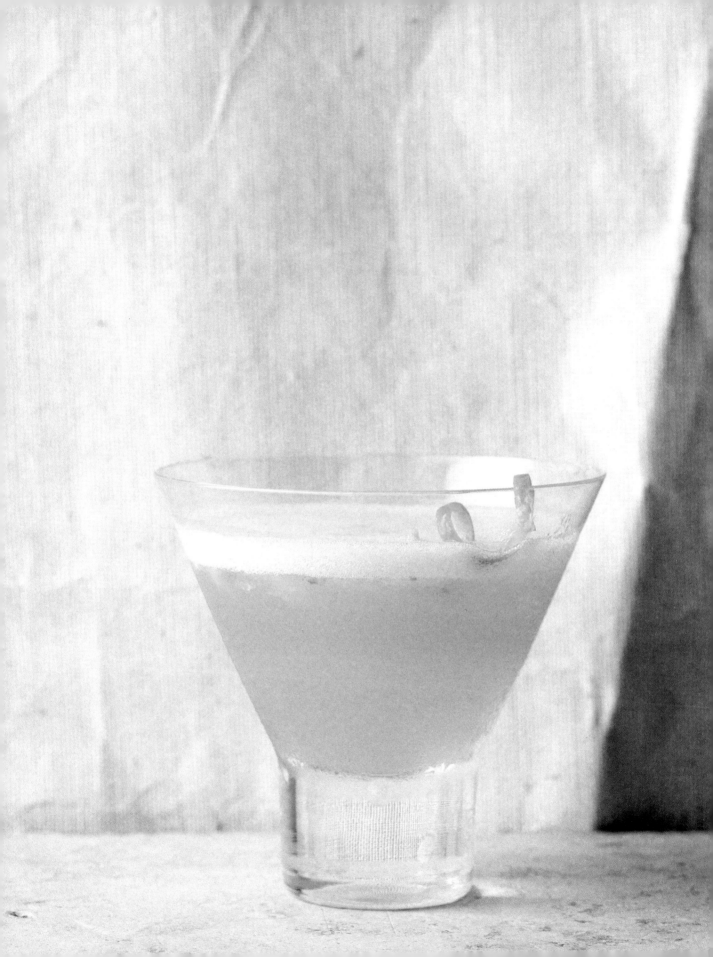

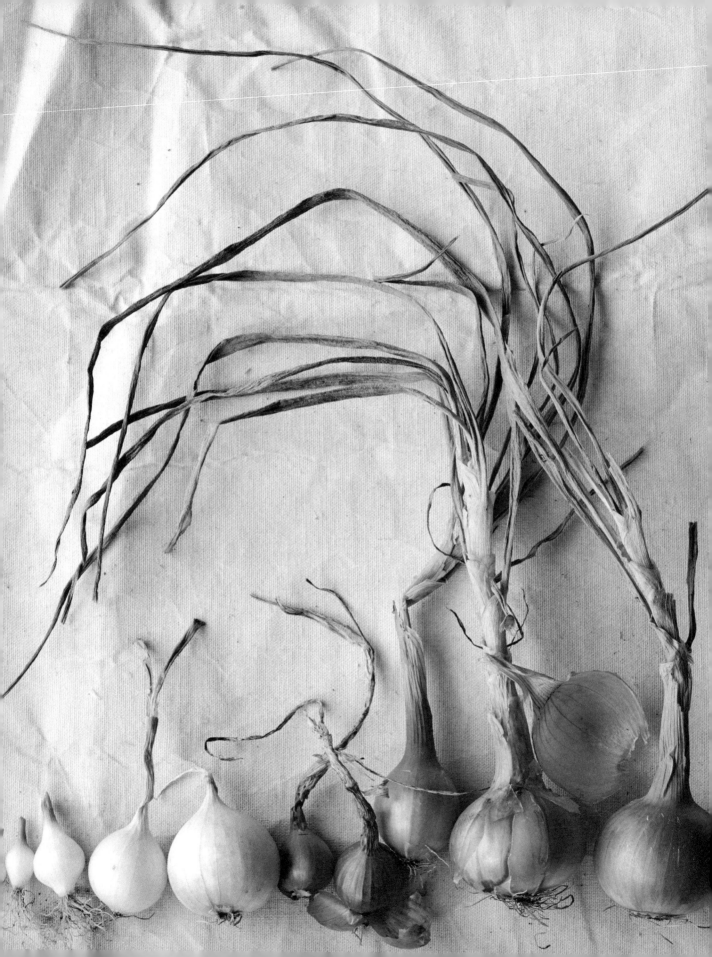

Basics

The recipes in this section are for sauces, stocks, spice mixtures, and condiments that are called for in the previous chapters and are good to have on hand. Many can be stored in the refrigerator or freezer to make your life in the kitchen easier. Knowing that I have a jar of fresh horseradish in my refrigerator makes me happy. With a supply of French vinaigrette, I can prepare a terrific green salad in a few minutes. I turn to dukkah and shichimi to liven up many foods. All of the recipes here are quick and easy. You will find that making these basics is well worth it.

Recipes marked **veg** are vegetarian, those marked **v** are vegan, and those marked **gf** are gluten-free. The symbols **veg***, **v***, and **gf*** indicate recipes that can be modified to be vegetarian, vegan, or gluten-free by substituting or omitting specific ingredients.

DASHI

MAKES 7 TO 8 CUPS, **GF**

Dashi is the universal broth used as a base for soups and sauces in Japanese cuisine. It derives its deep umami flavor from kombu (kelp), dried bonito flakes (available online or from Asian grocery stores), and shiitake mushrooms.

2 ounces dried shiitake mushroom caps

1 (20-inch-square) piece kombu

½ cup bonito flakes

1 tablespoon evaporated cane sugar

¼ cup low-sodium soy sauce

1. Put 2 quarts of water, the shiitake, and kombu in a large pot and bring to a boil. Cook over medium heat for 20 minutes, skimming off foam as necessary. Remove the kombu. Reduce the heat to a simmer and cook for 45 minutes.

2. Remove from the heat and whisk in the bonito flakes and sugar. Let the stock cool for 20 minutes. Strain through a fine-mesh sieve and discard the solids. Stir in the soy sauce. Transfer to lidded containers and refrigerate for up to 3 days or freeze for up to 1 month.

QUICK VEGETABLE STOCK

MAKES ABOUT 4 QUARTS, **V, GF**

Sweet potato and kombu provide umami flavor to this all-purpose stock. If you want more of that savory taste, add some shiitake mushrooms (fresh or dried). If the carrots and sweet potatoes are organic, you needn't peel them.

5 unpeeled garlic cloves, crushed

3 celery stalks, cut into large chunks

4 carrots, cut into large chunks

1 large unpeeled yellow onion, quartered

1 sweet potato, cut into large chunks

¼ cup fresh flat-leaf parsley leaves

6 peppercorns

1 Turkish bay leaf or ⅓ of a California bay leaf

1 (8-inch) strip kombu

1 teaspoon sea salt

1. Toss everything except the salt into an 8-quart pot filled with 4½ quarts (18 cups) of water, cover, and bring to a boil over high heat. Reduce the heat to medium-high for a brisk simmer and cook for 30 minutes with the lid slightly ajar. Turn off the heat and let the vegetables steep until the pot is cool enough to handle, about 30 minutes.

2. Strain the stock over a large bowl and stir in the salt. Transfer to pint and quart containers to freeze for future use. It will keep for up to 6 months.

BASIC FRENCH VINAIGRETTE

MAKES ABOUT ⅔ CUP, **V, GF**

This is my idea of a perfect salad dressing. You can vary it by adding finely chopped fresh dill, parsley, chervil, or tarragon. Use a Dijon mustard imported from France.

½ tablespoon real Dijon mustard

¼ teaspoon sea salt

½ tablespoon freshly squeezed lemon juice

½ tablespoon red or white wine vinegar

⅓ to ½ cup extra-virgin olive oil

Freshly ground black pepper, to taste

½ tablespoon finely minced shallot or scallion (white part only)

1. Put all the ingredients except the shallot or scallion in a jar and emulsify them with an immersion blender. Mix in the shallot or scallion.

2. Taste the dressing (dip a salad green into it) and adjust with salt, pepper, or drops of lemon juice, if necessary.

NOTE: The traditional mixing method is to stir the shallots or scallions together with the mustard and salt, whisk in the lemon juice and vinegar, and then, when well blended, whisk in the oil by droplets to form a smooth emulsion, adding the freshly ground pepper at the end, but it's easier to blend everything together in a jar with the solid disk of an immersion blender. You can also shake the ingredients vigorously in a jar, but that will not give you a true emulsion.

BASIC LEMON VINAIGRETTE

MAKES ½ CUP, **V, GF**

This is the simplest and yet most versatile vinaigrette and is used as the base for many of the salads in this book. All you need is a lemon and good-quality extra-virgin olive oil. Drizzle this on top of just about everything for a bright flavor pop. I often double this recipe in order to keep some in my refrigerator at all times.

1 teaspoon grated lemon zest

3 tablespoons lemon juice

½ teaspoon sea salt

½ teaspoon freshly ground black pepper

¼ cup extra-virgin olive oil

Whisk all the ingredients together in a small bowl, whisking in the oil last in a thin stream. Transfer to a lidded container. (Or use an immersion blender right in the container.) Store in the refrigerator for up to a week.

VARIATIONS:

Add 1 tablespoon of your favorite chopped herbs.

Add ½ teaspoon ground cumin for Lentil Tabbouleh (page 95).

Add 1 garlic clove, pressed and allowed to sit for 10 minutes, along with 1 tablespoon fresh oregano or 2 teaspoons dried whole oregano for Greek-Style Kale Salad (page 88).

Add ⅛ teaspoon ground coriander for Lemony Fennel Slaw (page 99).

Add 1 garlic clove, pressed and allowed to sit for 10 minutes, 1 teaspoon Dijon mustard, 1 small diced shallot, and 1 additional tablespoon of extra-virgin olive oil for Warm Mushroom Salad (page 114).

Add a generous pinch of crushed red pepper flakes for Zucchini Ribbons with Basil and Parmesan (page 140).

PREPARED FRESH HORSERADISH

MAKES ABOUT 2 CUPS, **V**, **GF**

This is a fabulous condiment that totally outclasses the stuff you buy in jars. Horseradish roots are available in the produce sections of many good supermarkets in most months of the year. Avoid ones that appear soft, shrunken, or dry. Cut off as much as you want to prepare and keep the remainder for later use in a storage bag in the crisper drawer of the refrigerator. The fumes from the freshly grated root are as irritating to the eyes, nose, and respiratory passages as tear gas; be careful not to inhale them. (I remember my grandmother grating horseradish by hand, tears streaming down her face. She would have been in awe of a food processor.) Once you add vinegar, the danger is past.

1 (8-inch-long, 2-inch-diameter) piece of horseradish root, peeled and cut into small pieces
1 tablespoon white vinegar
Pinch of sea salt

1. Place the horseradish in a food processor and process until well ground. Add the vinegar and salt and pulse to combine.

2. Using a spatula, carefully transfer the grated horseradish to a jar with a tight-fitting lid. It will keep for up to a month in the refrigerator.

GINGER-GARLIC STIR-FRY SAUCE

MAKES ½ CUP, **V**, **GF**

You can make enough of this flavorful sauce for a few stir-fries. Store it in the refrigerator for up to several days and shake well before use. Add it to a hot skillet when stir-fry ingredients are a few minutes from done, and let most of it evaporate before removing the pan from the heat.

2 garlic cloves, pressed and allowed to sit for 10 minutes
¼ cup low-sodium soy sauce
2 tablespoons lime juice
1½ tablespoons grade B maple syrup
1 tablespoon unseasoned rice vinegar
2 teaspoons minced or grated peeled ginger
Pinch of cayenne pepper

In a medium bowl whisk the ingredients together. Pour into a lidded container and refrigerate until ready to use.

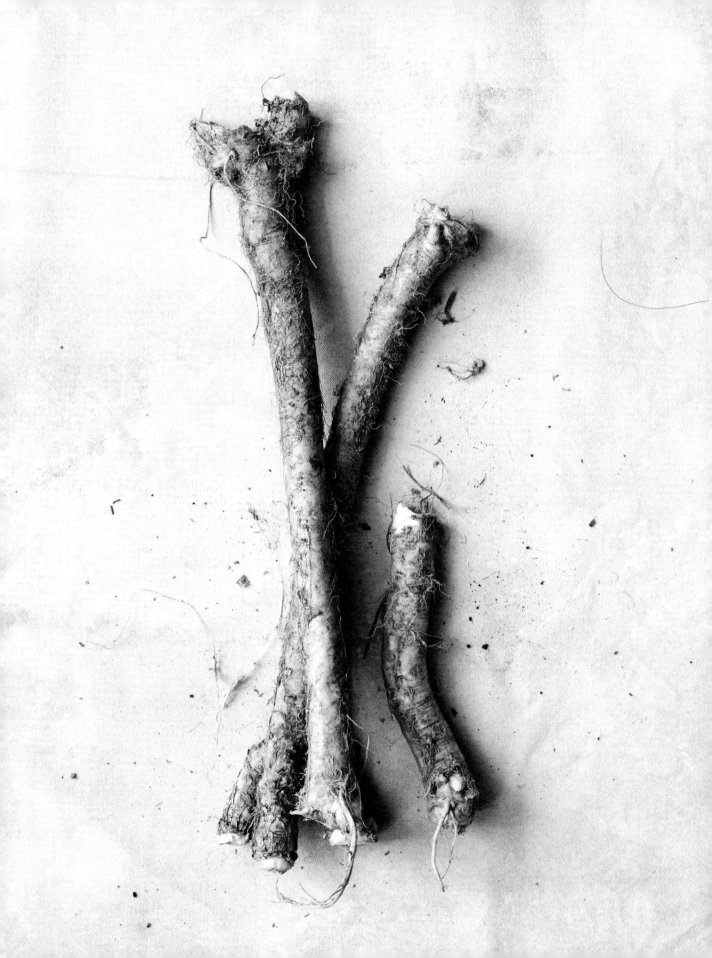

KALE PISTACHIO PESTO
with **GARLIC SCAPES**

MAKES 1½ CUPS, **V**, **GF**

Garlic scapes are the green flower stalks of hardneck garlic, available in spring. They keep for a long time and are delicious. If you can't find them, substitute 3 pressed garlic cloves and 3 tablespoons of chopped chives. You can enjoy this yummy pesto on vegetables and fish or on crackers. Or just lick it off your fingers.

4 to 5 large leaves black (lacinato, Tuscan) kale, stemmed

½ cup raw, unsalted pistachios

5 to 6 garlic scapes, flower buds removed, coarsely chopped

1 small bunch basil, leaves picked

Sea salt, to taste

½ cup extra-virgin olive oil

1. Steam the kale until just wilted and bright green. Let cool, squeeze out as much liquid as you can, and chop coarsely.

2. Grind the pistachios fine in a food processor. Add the garlic scapes, kale, basil, and salt and process to a coarse paste. Add the oil slowly with the motor running. If necessary, add a bit more oil to get the consistency you want.

3. Use as a spread or topping. For a pasta sauce, mix with freshly grated Parmesan cheese. The pesto keeps in the refrigerator in an airtight container for up to a week.

MISO BUTTER

MAKES ABOUT ½ CUP, **VEG**, **GF**

This compound butter is great on vegetables and fish. (Try it on steamed corn on the cob.) If you like it as much as I do, make a larger quantity and keep it in the refrigerator or freezer.

8 tablespoons unsalted butter

4 teaspoons white (shiro) miso

4 teaspoons lime juice

Mix all the ingredients together until well combined. Store in an airtight container in the refrigerator or freezer for up to 1 month.

WASABI BUTTER

MAKES ABOUT ¾ CUP, **VEG, GF**

Try a bit of this zippy compound butter on vegetables or fish.

4 tablespoons wasabi powder

8 tablespoons butter

4 teaspoons lime juice

½ teaspoon sea salt

Combine the wasabi powder in a small bowl with 2 tablespoons of water to make a paste. Mix in the remaining ingredients until well combined. Store in an airtight container in the refrigerator or freezer for up to a month.

QUICK PICKLED ONIONS

MAKES ABOUT 1 CUP, **V, GF**

This simple recipe makes a great garnish and is wonderful in salads. You will want to keep a supply on hand.

½ cup unseasoned rice vinegar

1 teaspoon evaporated cane sugar

Pinch of sea salt

1 red onion, thinly sliced

1. In a small bowl, combine the rice vinegar, sugar, and salt. Stir until dissolved.

2. Place the onions in a strainer. Slowly pour 2 cups of boiling water over the onions and shake the strainer to be sure all the onions are rinsed.

3. Toss the onions in the vinegar mixture while they are still warm. Let sit for at least 10 minutes, stirring periodically. They can be stored in an airtight container in the refrigerator for up to 2 weeks.

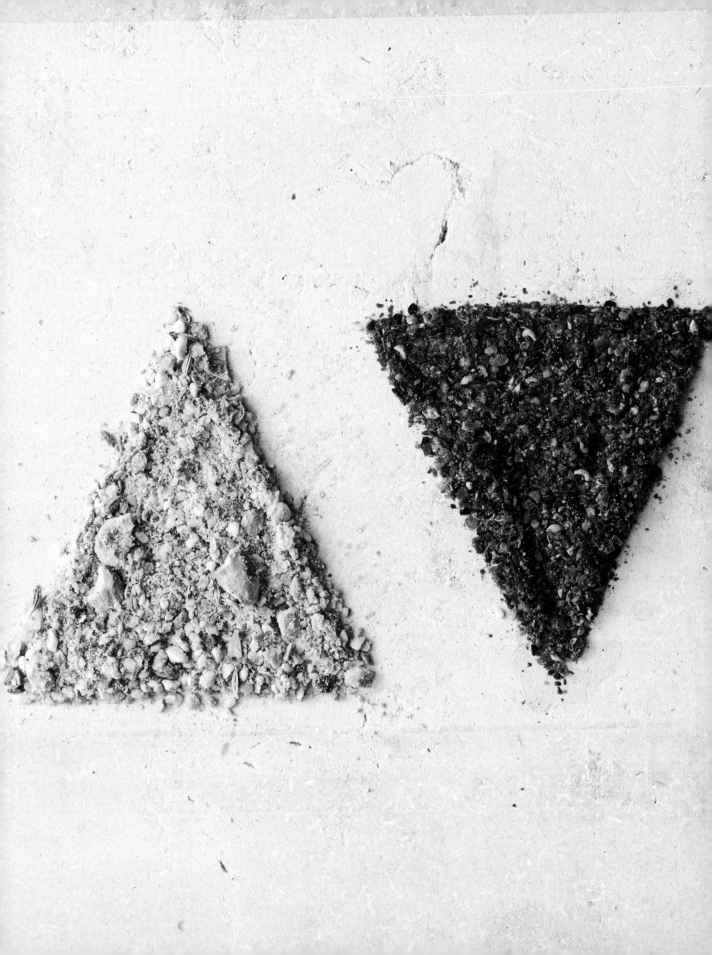

DUKKAH (MIDDLE EASTERN SPICE MIXTURE)

MAKES 1 CUP, **V, GF**

In Egypt, where this traditional spice blend originated, dukkah is made with hazelnuts. In this version, pistachios take their place, providing great taste, texture, and color. You can sprinkle it on everything, including vegetables, fish, dips, and toasted pita. Warning: addictive.

½ cup raw, unsalted pistachios

2 tablespoons raw white sesame seeds

1 tablespoon whole coriander seeds

1 tablespoon whole cumin seeds

2 teaspoons fennel seeds

¼ teaspoon sea salt

¼ teaspoon freshly ground black pepper

1. Heat a medium pan over medium heat and toast the pistachios until they are fragrant, about 3 minutes. Remove the pistachios from the pan and allow them to cool. Turn the heat down to low and add the sesame seeds, coriander, cumin, and fennel seeds. Toast until aromatic, about 2 minutes.

2. Place the pistachios in a food processor with a fitted blade and pulse until they reach the consistency of sand. Add the sesame seeds, coriander, cumin, and fennel and process until well blended. Transfer the mixture to a bowl and stir in the salt and pepper.

3. Store in an airtight container in the refrigerator for up to 1 month.

SHICHIMI

MAKES ½ CUP, **V, GF**

Shichimi, or "seven spice," is a universal Japanese seasoning, found in orange-capped shakers on the tables of many Japanese restaurants. It is fragrant and spicy and good on just about anything. Making it yourself is fun.

2 tablespoons Sichuan peppercorns

2 tablespoons crushed red pepper flakes

2 teaspoons hemp seeds

2 teaspoons dried ground orange peel

2 teaspoons ground ginger

½ sheet nori

2 tablespoons black sesame seeds, toasted

1½ teaspoons sea salt

1. Put the first six ingredients in a spice grinder or small food processor and pulse until the mixture is coarsely ground.

2. Stir in the sesame seeds and salt. Store in an airtight container for up to 3 months.

TOASTED NUTS AND SEEDS

Due to their high oil content and the fact that they continue to cook after being removed from the heat source, nuts can quickly turn from perfectly toasted to burned. A general rule is that once you can smell the nuts, they are done.

1. To toast nuts and seeds on the stovetop: Spread a single layer of raw nuts in a dry skillet and set over medium heat. Move the nuts around the pan, turning them over every minute or two. When you can smell the nuts and they begin to color, transfer them to a plate to cool.

2. To toast nuts (including coconut) in the oven: Preheat the oven to 350°F and line a rimmed baking sheet with parchment paper. Spread a single layer of raw nuts on the baking sheet and bake for 8 to 12 minutes, turning them once halfway through cooking.

3. Toasted nuts quickly go rancid, so use them up soon after preparing them or store them in a zip-top bag in the freezer for up to a month.

CROUTONS OR BREAD CRUMBS

MAKES ABOUT 3 CUPS, **V**

The big advantage of making your own croutons is that you have control of the quality of bread and oil you are using. Croutons can easily be made into rustic bread crumbs, which are perfect for the dishes in this book. Croutons and bread crumbs can be stored in zip-top bags in the freezer for up to 6 months.

4 slices day-old (or older) whole-grain bread, cut into ½-inch cubes

2 teaspoons extra-virgin olive oil

¼ teaspoon sea salt

Freshly ground black pepper

1. Preheat the oven to 350°F and line a baking sheet with parchment paper.

2. Toss the bread cubes with olive oil, salt, and a few grinds of freshly ground black pepper.

3. Spread them evenly on the baking sheet and bake for 10 to 15 minutes, stirring occasionally, until they're golden and crispy. Remove from the oven and allow them to cool.

4. To make bread crumbs, pulse the cooled croutons in a food processor about 15 times or until they are coarsely ground. Overprocessing may result in a sandy texture or paste.

CASHEW MILK

MAKES 3 CUPS, **V, GF**

I find cashew milk to be the perfect substitute for milk or cream in soups, sauces, and desserts. You can make it rich or lean by varying the ratio of nuts to water. The 1 to 2 ratio below approximates the richness of whole milk.
I prefer to use whole raw cashews, as they are of better quality than broken ones. You will want to keep some of this on hand; it will hold in the refrigerator for up to 10 days.

1 cup raw whole cashews

1. Grind the cashews to a fine powder in a blender or food processor, stopping and stirring occasionally to ensure uniform grinding. Depending on the machine you use, this will take 1 to 3 minutes. Stop before the nuts turn into a paste.

2. Add 2 cups of room-temperature water, blend on medium speed for 30 seconds, and then stop and stir up any nuts that stick to the sides of the container. Blend on high speed for 2 minutes. Store in an airtight container in the refrigerator for up to 10 days. Shake well before using.

MAPLE SIMPLE SYRUP

MAKES 1¾ CUPS, **V, GF**

Most simple syrups are made with refined white sugar. I suggest using organic maple syrup instead. (It has a lower content of fructose and some trace minerals.) Use grade A for clear drinks and the more rustic grade B for darker drinks. As with all sweeteners, use sparingly.

¾ cup grade A maple syrup

Combine the maple syrup with 1 cup of water in a saucepan over medium heat. Bring to a boil, then turn off heat and allow to cool. Transfer to a lidded jar and refrigerate until needed. It will keep for up to 10 days.

MAPLE CINNAMON
SIMPLE SYRUP

MAKES ¾ CUP, **V**, **GF**

3 ounces grade A maple syrup

2 cinnamon sticks, broken into 2-inch lengths

In a small saucepan, combine the maple syrup and ½ cup water. Add the cinnamon sticks. Bring to a boil and simmer for about 5 minutes over low heat. Remove from the heat and allow to cool with the cinnamon in the pan. Remove the sticks. Transfer syrup to a lidded jar and refrigerate until needed. It will keep for up to 10 days.

SPEARMINT OR BASIL
SIMPLE SYRUP

MAKES 1¾ CUPS, **V**, **GF**

Many cocktail recipes call for simple syrup, which is made with sugar and water, but simple syrup can easily be infused with other flavors. Two of my favorites are fresh spearmint and fresh basil. Both add a new level of interest to margaritas, daiquiris, and other refreshing summer drinks.

¾ cup grade A maple syrup

1 cup loosely packed basil or spearmint leaves

Combine the maple syrup, basil or spearmint leaves, and 1 cup of water in a saucepan over medium heat. Bring to a boil. Turn off the heat and allow to cool. After 10 minutes, strain the leaves. Transfer the syrup to a lidded jar and refrigerate until needed. It will keep for up to 10 days.

GINGER-SPEARMINT SYRUP

MAKES 2 CUPS, **V**, **GF**

Another lovely flavored syrup that can enhance both alcoholic and nonalcoholic drinks.

2 cups peeled and sliced ginger (about 1 "hand")

24 spearmint leaves, plus sprigs for serving

2 tablespoons lime juice

2 tablespoons grade B maple syrup

1. Bring 4 cups of water, the ginger, and the spearmint leaves to a boil in a saucepan, then lower the heat to medium and simmer uncovered for 20 to 30 minutes or until the liquid has reduced by half.

2. Strain the infusion into a quart-size mason jar and discard the ginger and spearmint leaves. Stir in the lime juice and maple syrup and let cool to room temperature. This mixture can be kept in the refrigerator for up to 2 weeks or frozen for 3 months.

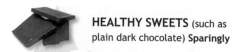

HEALTHY SWEETS (such as plain dark chocolate) **Sparingly**

RED WINE (optional)
No more than 1-2 glasses a day

SUPPLEMENTS
Daily

TEA (white, green, oolong)
2-4 cups a day

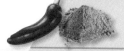

HEALTHY HERBS & SPICES (such as garlic, ginger, turmeric, cinnamon) **Unlimited amounts**

OTHER SOURCES OF PROTEIN (dairy [natural cheeses, yogurt], omega-3 enriched eggs, skinless poultry, lean meats) **1-2 a week**

COOKED ASIAN MUSHROOMS
Unlimited amounts

WHOLE SOY FOODS (edamame, soy nuts, soymilk, tofu, tempeh) **1-2 a day**

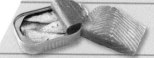

FISH & SHELLFISH (wild Alaskan salmon, Alaskan black cod, sardines) **2-6 a week**

HEALTHY FATS (extra-virgin olive oil, nuts—especially walnuts, avocados, seeds—including hemp seeds and freshly ground flaxseeds) **5-7 a day**

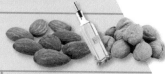

WHOLE & CRACKED GRAINS 3-5 a day	**PASTA (al dente)** 2-3 a week	**BEANS & LEGUMES** 1-2 a day

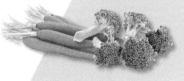

VEGETABLES (both raw and cooked, from all parts of the color spectrum, organic when possible) **4-5 a day minimum**

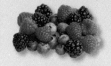

FRUITS (fresh in season or frozen, organic when possible) **3-4 a day**

THE ANTI-INFLAMMATORY DIET
AND PYRAMID

The Anti-Inflammatory Diet is not a diet in the popular sense—it is not intended as a weight-loss program (although people can and do lose weight on it), nor is it an eating plan to stay on for a limited time. Rather, it is a way of selecting and preparing foods based on scientific knowledge of how they can help your body maintain optimum health. Along with decreasing inflammation, this diet will provide you with steady energy and ample vitamins, minerals, essential fatty acids, dietary fiber, and protective phytonutrients.

HEALTHY SWEETS

How much: Sparingly

Healthy choices: Unsweetened dried fruit, dark chocolate, fruit sorbet

Why: Dark chocolate provides polyphenols with antioxidant activity. Choose dark chocolate with at least 70 percent pure cacao and have an ounce a few times a week. Fruit sorbet is a better option than other frozen desserts.

RED WINE

How much: Optional, no more than 1 to 2 glasses per day

Healthy choices: Organic red wine

Why: Red wine has beneficial antioxidant activity. Limit intake to no more than 1 to 2 servings per day. If you do not drink alcohol, do not start.

SUPPLEMENTS

How much: Daily

Healthy choices: High-quality multivitamin/ multimineral that includes key antioxidants (vitamin C, vitamin E, mixed carotenoids, and selenium); coenzyme Q10; 2 to 3 grams of a molecularly distilled fish oil; 2,000 IU of vitamin D3

Why: Supplements help fill gaps in your diet when you are unable to get your daily requirement of micronutrients.

TEA

How much: 2 to 4 cups per day

Healthy choices: White, green, oolong teas

Why: Tea is rich in catechins, antioxidant compounds that reduce inflammation. Purchase high-quality tea and learn how to brew it correctly for maximum taste and health benefits.

HEALTHY HERBS AND SPICES

How much: Unlimited amounts

Healthy choices: Turmeric, curry powder (which contains turmeric), ginger and garlic (dried and fresh), chili peppers, basil, cinnamon, rosemary, thyme

Why: Use these herbs and spices generously to season foods. Turmeric and ginger are powerful natural anti-inflammatory agents.

OTHER SOURCES OF PROTEIN

How much: 1 to 2 servings a week (one portion is equal to 1 ounce of cheese, one 8-ounce serving of dairy, 1 egg, or 3 ounces cooked poultry or skinless meat)

Healthy choices: High-quality natural cheese and yogurt, omega-3-enriched eggs, skinless poultry, grass-finished lean meats

Why: In general, try to reduce consumption of animal foods. If you eat chicken, choose organic, cage-free chicken and remove the skin and associated fat. Use organic dairy products moderately, primarily yogurt and natural cheeses such as Emmental (Swiss), Jarlsberg, and true Parmesan. If you eat eggs, choose omega-3-enriched eggs (from hens that are fed a flax-meal-enriched diet) or organic eggs from free-range chickens.

COOKED ASIAN MUSHROOMS

How much: Unlimited amounts

Healthy choices: Shiitake, enokitake, maitake, oyster mushrooms (and wild mushrooms if available)

Why: These mushrooms contain compounds that enhance immune function. Never eat mushrooms raw, and minimize consumption of common commercial button mushrooms (including cremini and Portobello).

WHOLE-SOY FOODS

How much: 1 to 2 servings per day (one serving is equal to ½ cup tofu or tempeh, 1 cup soy milk, ½ cup cooked edamame, or 1 ounce of soy nuts)

Healthy choices: Tofu, tempeh, edamame, soy nuts, soy milk

Why: Soy foods contain isoflavones that have antioxidant activity and are protective against cancer. Choose whole-soy foods over fractionated foods like isolated soy-protein powders and imitation meats made with soy isolate.

FISH AND SHELLFISH

How much: 2 to 6 servings per week (one serving is equal to 4 ounces of fish or seafood)

Healthy choices: Wild Alaskan salmon (especially sockeye), herring, sardines, and black cod (sablefish)

Why: These fish are rich in omega-3 fats, which are strongly anti-inflammatory. If you choose not to eat fish, take a molecularly distilled fish-oil supplement that provides both EPA and DHA in a dose of 2 to 3 grams per day.

HEALTHY FATS

How much: 5 to 7 servings per day (one serving is equal to 1 teaspoon of oil, 2 walnuts, 1 tablespoon of flaxseed, 1 ounce of avocado)

Healthy choices: For cooking, use extra-virgin olive oil and expeller-pressed grapeseed oil. Other sources of healthy fats are nuts (especially walnuts), avocados, and seeds, including hemp seeds and freshly ground flaxseed. Omega-3 fats are also found in cold-water fish, omega-3-enriched eggs, and whole-soy foods. Organic, expeller-pressed, high-oleic sunflower or safflower oils may also be used, as well as walnut and hazelnut oils in salads and dark roasted sesame oil as a flavoring for soups and stir-fries.

Why: Healthy fats are those rich in either monounsaturated or omega-3 fats. Extra-virgin olive oil is rich in polyphenols with antioxidant activity.

WHOLE AND CRACKED GRAINS

How much: 3 to 5 servings a day (one serving is equal to about ½ cup cooked grains)

Healthy choices: Brown rice, basmati rice, wild rice, buckwheat groats, barley, quinoa, steel-cut oats

Why: Whole grains digest slowly, reducing frequency of spikes in blood sugar that promote inflammation. *Whole grains* means grains that are intact or in a few large pieces, not whole-wheat bread or other products made from flour.

PASTA (AL DENTE)

How much: 2 to 3 servings per week (one serving is equal to about ½ cup cooked pasta)

Healthy choices: Organic pasta, rice noodles, bean thread noodles, and part whole-wheat and buckwheat noodles like Japanese udon and soba

Why: Pasta cooked al dente (when it has "tooth" to it) has a lower glycemic index than fully cooked pasta. Low-glycemic-load carbohydrates should be the bulk of your carbohydrate intake to help minimize spikes in blood glucose levels.

BEANS AND LEGUMES

How much: 1 to 2 servings per day (one serving is equal to ½ cup cooked beans or legumes)

Healthy choices: Beans like Anasazi, adzuki, and black beans, as well as chickpeas, black-eyed peas, and lentils

Why: Beans are rich in folic acid, magnesium, potassium, and soluble fiber. They are a low-glycemic-load food. Eat them well cooked either whole or pureed in spreads like hummus.

VEGETABLES

How much: 4 to 5 servings per day minimum (one serving is equal to 2 cups salad greens or ½ cup vegetables cooked, raw, or juiced)

The Anti-Inflammatory Diet and Pyramid

Healthy choices: Lightly cooked dark leafy greens (spinach, collard greens, kale, Swiss chard), cruciferous vegetables (broccoli, cabbage, Brussels sprouts, kale, bok choy, and cauliflower), carrots, beets, onions, peas, squashes, sea vegetables, and washed raw salad greens

Why: Vegetables are rich in flavonoids and carotenoids with both antioxidant and anti-inflammatory activity. Go for a wide range of colors, eat them both raw and cooked, and choose organic when possible.

FRUITS

How much: 3 to 4 servings per day (one serving is equal to 1 medium-size piece of fruit, ½ cup chopped fruit, ½ cup of dried fruit)

Healthy choices: Raspberries, blueberries, strawberries, peaches, nectarines, oranges, pink grapefruit, red grapes, plums, pomegranates, blackberries, cherries, apples, and pears—all lower in glycemic load than most tropical fruits

Why: Fruits are rich in flavonoids and carotenoids with both antioxidant and anti-inflammatory activity. Go for a wide range of colors, choose fruit that is fresh in season or frozen, and buy organic when possible.

WATER

How much: Throughout the day

Healthy choices: Drink pure water, or drinks that are mostly water (tea, very diluted fruit juice, sparkling water with lemon) throughout the day.

Why: Water is vital for overall functioning of the body.

ACKNOWLEDGMENTS

I thank my editor at Little, Brown, Tracy Behar; my agent Richard Pine; my business partner, Richard Baxter; and my executive assistant, Nancy Olmstead, for their help in making this book possible. Working with them is always rewarding.

Producing a cookbook involves a lot of attention to detail. I could not have done this one without the assistance of a great team. First and foremost, I am indebted to my friend and colleague Rebecca Katz, a skilled chef and author of a number of excellent cookbooks who provided, vetted, and tested recipes, turned me on to ingredients and techniques new to me, and organized the manuscript with great proficiency. She, in turn, wishes to thank her colleagues Catherine McConkie and Jen Yasis for helping her with recipe testing, as well as her canine companions, Bella and Lola, who cleaned up scraps. Rebecca and I love to cook and teach together, and I look forward to more collaborations with her.

Dr. Jim Nicolai helped me test and refine recipes, as did Stacy Wrona, a chef in Tucson. Jeanie Linders provided a test kitchen that we put to good use. Jonathan Heindemause contributed recipes and ideas to the book, as did Kengo Ikeda, Paul Remer, Julie Burford, Nori Fletcher, and Stacy Wrona.

Ditte Isager of New York and Copenhagen, with whom I have worked before, did the outstanding photography in these pages. I am grateful that she made time in her busy schedule to do so; it is an invaluable addition.

Christine Rudolph was the prop stylist and Susie Theodorou the food stylist for the book.

Finally, I thank my own canine assistant, Ajax, who put his stamp of approval on most of the recipes and lent his name to one.

index

Page numbers in *italic* refer to photographs.

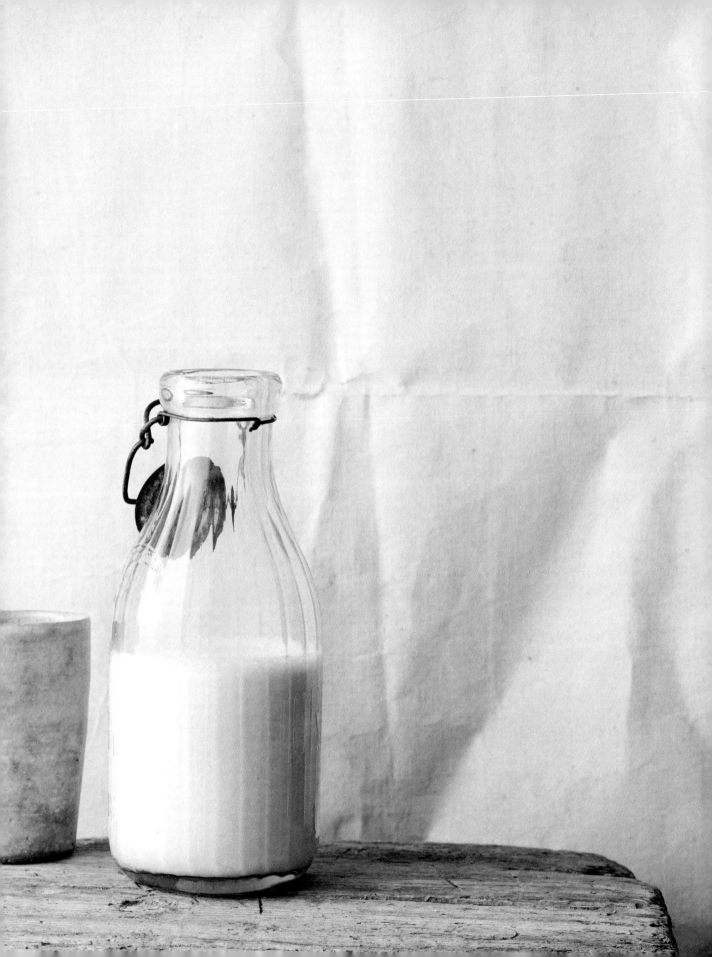

ABOUT THE AUTHOR

ANDREW WEIL, MD, is a world-renowned leader and pioneer in the field of integrative medicine, a healing-oriented approach to health care that encompasses body, mind, and spirit.

Dr. Weil is the founder and director of the Arizona Center for Integrative Medicine at the University of Arizona Health Sciences Center, where he is also a clinical professor of medicine, professor of public health, and the Lovell-Jones Professor of Integrative Rheumatology. Dr. Weil received both his medical degree and his undergraduate degree in biology (botany) from Harvard University.

Dr. Weil is an internationally recognized expert on maintaining a healthy lifestyle, healthy aging, and the future of medicine and health care. Approximately ten million copies of Dr. Weil's books have been sold, among them *True Food, Spontaneous Happiness, Spontaneous Healing, Eight Weeks to Optimum Health, Eating Well for Optimum Health, The Healthy Kitchen*, and *Healthy Aging*.

He is the editorial director of drweil.com, the leading Web resource for healthy living based on the philosophy of integrative medicine. He authors the popular "Self-Healing" newsletter and special publications. As a columnist for *Prevention* magazine and a frequent guest on numerous national shows, Dr. Weil provides valuable insight and information on how to incorporate conventional and complementary medicine practices into one's life to optimize the body's natural healing power.

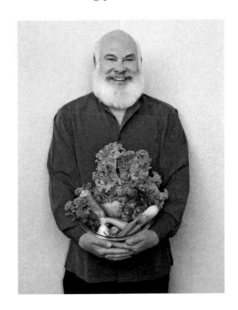